HEALING
MUDRAS

Yoga for Your Hands

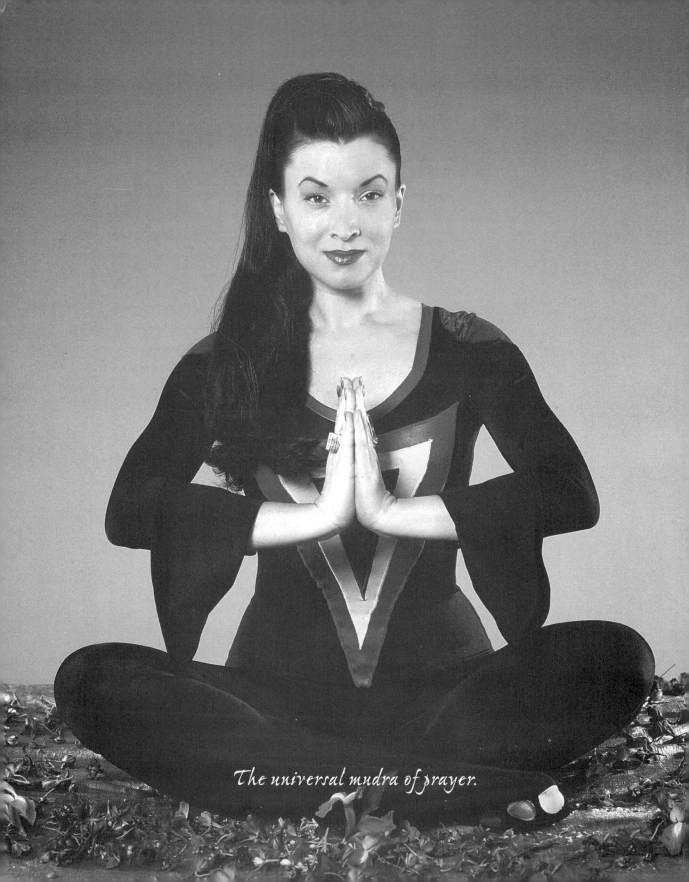

The universal mudra of prayer.

HEALING
MUDRAS

Yoga for Your Hands

Sabrina Mesko

Ballantine Wellspring™

The Ballantine Publishing Group • New York

A Ballantine Wellspring™ Book
Published by The Ballantine Publishing Group

Copyright © 2000 by Sabrina Mesko

Photography by Dorothy Low
Illustrations by Kiar Mesko
Costume design, photo design, and styling by Sabrina Mesko

All rights reserved under International
and Pan-American Copyright Conventions. Published
in the United States by The Ballantine Publishing Group, a division
of Random House, Inc., New York, and simultaneously in
Canada by Random House of Canada Limited, Toronto.
Based on an edition that was self-published
in 1997 under the title *The Yoga Dance.*

Ballantine is a registered trademark and Ballantine Wellspring and
the Ballantine Wellspring colophon are trademarks of Random House, Inc.

www.randomhouse.com/BB/wellspring/

Library of Congress Catalog Card Number: 99-91635

ISBN 0-345-43758-6

Cover design by Barbara Leff
Cover photo by Dorothy Low
Text design by Holly Johnson

Manufactured in the United States of America

First Ballantine Edition: February 2000

10   9   8   7   6   5   4   3

To the greatest parents in the world,
Bibi and Kiar

Contents

Acknowledgments

This book manifested in my hands through divine hands. Now this book and its energy are yours. I thank the Divine Universe for giving me the opportunity to help others.

My deepest gratitude to the following wonderful people:

I must thank my teachers, gurus, and masters whom I learned from and had the privilege to meet: Guru Maya, Paramahansa Yogananda, Bhikram, Sri Sri Ravi Shankar, and, most of all, Yogi Bhajan.

My parents, Kiar and Bibi, who sacrificed much, and encouraged and guided me on my life's journey. I love you.

My brother, Kristopher, and sister, Iris, for their support.

My agent, Lisa Swayne, for her belief and guidance from the start.

My editor, Leslie Meredith, for her vision and for recognizing the beauty, power, and importance of these hand teachings.

And Jeff Kutash—the angel protector—for his extraordinary love and encouragement every day in every way.

Thank you all from the bottom of my heart and soul.

Love and peace and blessings.

HEALING
MUDRAS

Yoga for Your Hands

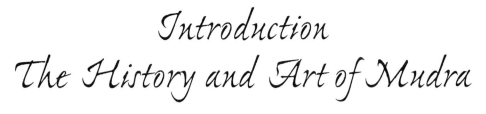

Introduction
The History and Art of Mudra

My journey to create this book has been a long but inspiring one. It has undoubtedly taken me quite a few lifetimes to achieve it. I believe that we all have a mission in our life that we have chosen to accomplish—even before we are born. This book is mine.

Finding your life's purpose can be quite a challenge. You may think you know why you are here and what you are supposed to do with your life. Yet an event or a series of events can uproot you, whirl you completely around, and deposit you on a completely new path. Astoundingly, we often find that this path is the one that we were looking for all along, even though it is not the path we had envisioned for ourselves.

I grew up in Ljubljana in Slovenia, in an enormously talented, artistic family. My father is an artist and sculptor, my mother a journalist and linguist. My sister, an archaeologist, has done extensive research on dance in Egypt, and my brother specializes in spiritual art. Every day of my early life, I was surrounded by love and an appreciation for beauty and saw all around me the profound and enlivening effect that art has on the enjoyment and quality of daily life. I was propelled into my love of dance and music even before I could really walk. I became a professional ballerina in my teens and danced in classical ballet companies all over Europe.

Because I have always had a tremendous desire to help people, I also taught disabled and blind children how to dance. This experience confirmed my belief that encouragement and positive feedback can make a great difference in our ability to face the challenges that life presents us. The world can seem a hard place, and it is very important to show each other and especially our younger generation that we can achieve our dreams, and that we can do so without compromising our beliefs or ourselves. I truly believe that there is a rewarding and positive answer to every problem that enters our lives. Our daily mission is to find that better way, pursue it ourselves, and open it to the next person behind us. Together, we can turn our world into a harmonious and happy one.

To be most effective in accomplishing our daily mission and our life's mission, and to deal effectively with life's challenges, we must first find an inner peace and strength within ourselves. The techniques presented in this book give you the key to unlocking the limitless powers that lie within you. You have been born with all the inner resources you need—you have only to discover and develop them. This book of mudras is a quick instruction guide to getting to know your sacred powers and freeing them for your use every day. Mudra is the password to the data of your inner computer—your unseen power. All you have to do is activate one function at a time—there is only one mudra on each page, so you can proceed at your own pace in this spiritual strength training—and you will discover a new way to re-program your body, mind, and soul to achieve your full potential.

I began to practice yoga after a back injury cut into my dancing career. Eventually, I realized that dance had been only the connecting path to my true life's mission of studying and teaching yoga—particularly yoga that you can use to help you live your daily life. Mudras are wonderfully effective—and easy to do—yet until now they have not been widely taught as a technique for living.

Even though I had studied different meditation teachings and techniques for many years, it took me a long time to develop a deep understanding of the hand gestures of mudras. Aside from a few very basic mudras used for common meditations, the hundred-plus mudras themselves just weren't being taught. For several years while studying yoga and holistic medicine, I couldn't find any information about mudras. I continued to search, however, and was fortunate to eventually meet wonderful teachers and masters who instructed me in the art of mudra. As the saying goes, when the student is ready, the master will appear. This certainly was true in my case. When I was ready for the next level of my training, events would unfold in such a way that I would be led to my next teacher. As I studied meditation, breathing, and yoga, I had the constant feeling that I was being reminded of something familiar rather than learning something completely new. When I finally began to practice mudra techniques for the first time, I instantly felt that my entire life journey made sense. Now it brings me great joy and a sense of fulfillment to share this knowledge and technique with you.

A Brief History

Hand gestures have been native to every culture on earth and can be seen as intrinsic to civilization: Ancient Egyptians, Romans, Greeks, Persians, Aborigines in Australia, ancient Indians and Chinese, Africans, Turks, Fijians, Mayan cultures, Inuit, and the Native American nations all used hand language.

Today, we still use hand language. Think about the universal handshake—a sign of friendship and peace. Applause is the language for approval and enthusiasm; the pointed index finger is used to scold; an upraised hand with the palm out signals us to stop.

There are many points of view regarding the development of hand gestures. Scientists have proved that even apes communicate with their hands and firmly believe that hand gestures were a basis for speech. A blind child who has never been able to see will still clap his hands to express excitement and happiness. Many hand gestures are universal, dating back thousands of years. In Egypt almost five thousand years ago, hand gestures were performed in prayer rituals by high priests and priestesses. Sacred hand gestures were key to communicating with the gods, manifesting miracles, and connecting with the afterlife. Egyptians carved these sacred gestures in bas-reliefs on the walls of and inside the pyramids, and they became the basis for their hieroglyphs. From Egypt, these movements and knowledge of their spiritual power and usage traveled to India and Greece.

In India, these gestures were named "mudras," a Sanskrit word, and they became an irreplaceable part of yoga, which aimed to connect the practitioner to divine and cosmic energy. Mudras became the essence of this divine communication in Buddhism and Hinduism. Buddhist priests developed the understanding of mudras still further and used them to close prayer rituals, a practice that has remained alive to this day. Plato placed hand gestures among the civil virtues in ancient Greece, where there was a distinct classification of hand gestures into comic, tragic, and satiric. From Egypt and Greece, these hand gestures were brought to Rome, where they became intrinsic to popular discourse and culture.

In the reign of Emperor Augustus in Rome, performances of hand gestures in pantomimic dances were a great personal delight of the emperor. Competitions were held between the best hand-gesture dancers, and all Rome was split into factions about their favorites. The most distinguished performer was often called the Dancing Philosopher.

A story from a later time in the Empire tells of the Armenian king visiting to pay his respects to Emperor Nero. Upon his departure, he was asked what he would most like to take home, and he replied, "The hand dancer, because he speaks better with hands than my people do with words."

In the year 190, there were six thousand performers in Rome devoted to the art of hand gesture. Their popularity continued until the sixth century A.D. Sacred hand gestures were also used in religious practice among Jews. In various portrayals of Moses we can observe him using mudras with gestures of blessing, divine protection, knowledge, and receiving guidance from the divine.

In Christianity, mudras took on a less noticeable form. Stylized hand poses are almost always present in portrayals of Jesus, but most people were not taught the significance of these poses. So the people in Western cultures lost the awareness of the healing and sacred power of the mudras and used them more as expressive communication gestures.

In Italian paintings before and during the Renaissance, one of the most common hand poses is that of the connected thumb and index finger. Its meaning is that the ego—the index finger—is bowing to God—the thumb—in love and unity. In popular Neapolitan use, that gesture is called the kissing of the thumb and finger—the sign of love. In secular portraits, that gesture translates into approval of love and marriage. Some Native Americans also used that hand gesture when indicating that they thought something was good and approved of it.

Another common gesture in religious paintings is that of the palm turned upward. This pose dates back centuries and signifies openness and inquiry. In this book, it is part of the mudra of asking for guidance, and it has a part in the mudra for facing fear (page 98). When you ask the universe to protect and guide you, the palm is held so that something can be placed in your hand—something can come to you. American Indians translated this gesture into: Give me!

A gesture in which the pointed index finger moves in a circle has a universal connection—specifically, "no"-rejection in Italian, Native American, and Japanese cultures, among others. When the index finger is pointed but motionless in popular usage and in high Italian art, it means indication, justice, pointing something out (which has led to the actual name of index for the forefinger). It can also mean silence, attention, number, mediation, and demonstration.

Native Americans were among the most famed hand-sign communicators, usually signing in front of strangers. Early white settlers actually believed that the American Indians rarely used spoken language, since the settlers most often saw them using hand gestures, but the Indians were of course simply being cautious and using hand gestures that Europeans didn't understand. Later on, Native Americans would play a key role in communicating with hearing-impaired children.

In Mexico, hand signs are found in elaborate ancient carvings, and they are also painted on ancient Greek and Homeric vases and pottery writings. The Chinese alphabet actually originated as the depiction of hand gestures. There are many commonalities among the hand gestures of Native American, Chinese, Egyptian, and African cultures. I hope that archaeologists, anthropologists, and linguists can eventually piece together how these universal gestures came to be used in such different parts of the world. Hand gestures are the mother of all communication and are supremely powerful. The art of mudra is divinely inspired: It enables us to communicate with the divine, develop and aspire to higher qualities, and keep a universally understood popular language. Mudra is our connection to the divine play of the cosmos.

The time has come to revive and appreciate the gift of mudra practice to utilize these efficient, powerful ancient techniques in everyday life. Mudra can help you follow your dreams: Your life is in your hands. This book is the manifestation of my dream of being of service. You are holding it in your hands, and I know from personal experience that mudras can help you achieve your best; heal your mind, body, and spirit; change your life for the better; and bring you to a new level of self-awareness and personal power.

I hope you will enjoy discovering the world of mudras and getting to know your own innate spiritual nature and gifts. Mudras will help you heal your soul and this world. I will remain eternally grateful for being given the opportunity to be the instrument for the transmission of these sacred teachings to you.

One in Spirit, love, and peace,

Sabrina

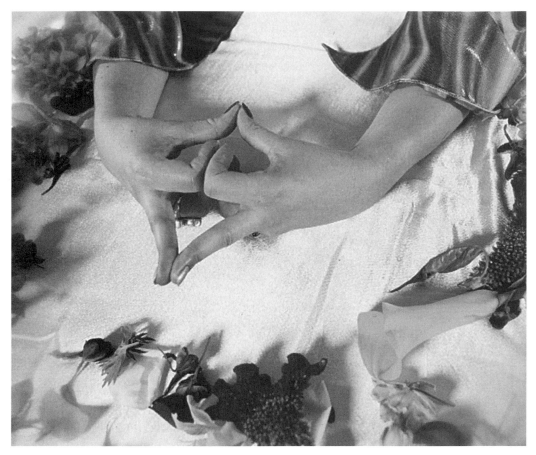

Mudra for tranquilizing the mind.

The Practice of Mudra

Instructions for Practice

Where do I practice mudra?

To practice mudra, find a quiet, peaceful, and private place where no one can disturb you. If that is not always possible, you can usually practice most of the mudras that are unobtrusive just about anywhere.

How do I practice mudra?

During the practice, it is best to sit in a comfortable position. You can sit on a pillow or blanket in a cross-legged position, or in a chair, but make sure your weight on both feet is equal. It is most important that you keep your back straight. Maintain a comfortable sitting posture that does *not* give you pain.

When should I practice mudra?

You can practice a mudra virtually any time that you feel the need to connect with the energy that it gives you. If you are practicing a mudra for insight or to enhance your meditation, however, the easiest time to concentrate is in the morning right after you wake up or in the evening before going to sleep. You should never practice a mudra on a full stomach, because your body-mind's energy is concentrated in your abdomen. Your overall energy is slow and needs to be permitted to be unimpeded as it focuses on turning nourishment into physical energy. After a meal, wait an hour before practice.

How often can I practice mudra?

You can practice as many mudras a day as you wish, but to obtain the full benefit that a mudra can give you, you will want to establish at least one three-minute set time during the day in which to grow comfortable with your mudra.

To feel the benefits faster, I recommend that you practice the mudra twice a day, each time for at least three minutes. Select a mudra that addresses a problem you have or a quality you want to develop, and make it a point to practice that mudra every day.

How long should I practice a mudra?

You should practice a mudra in the beginning for at least three minutes a day, but when you have built up your strength and ability to hold the mudra and evoke its energy, you can extend your practice to eleven minutes. Ultimately, you may want to build up your practice to thirty-one minutes once a day.

Most of the mudras will give you immediate results, in the form of more energy, clarity and peace of mind, or insight. More challenging or entrenched problems, however, will require more discipline and perseverance in your practice. It will take a few weeks of practice for the mudra to come into full effect and help you feel a profound transformation that will eliminate or resolve your problem.

Meditation

There are many different meditative techniques. If you have not meditated before, the simplest way to begin meditating is to find a quiet place and sit comfortably. Bring your attention to your breath: Exhale and inhale slowly through your nose and concentrate on your breath as it travels in and out of your body. As you concentrate, allow the awareness of your breath to still your mind and relax your body. You have begun to experience the essential state of meditation.

Meditation will lower your body temperature, so, when you plan to meditate for longer than eleven minutes, you should cover your back and shoulders with a shawl before sitting down.

With mudras and proper breathing, you can achieve deeper levels of meditation. You will experience peace, relaxation, rejuvenation, and higher levels of consciousness.

Your intuition, patience, and wisdom will increase greatly, as will your personal magnetism and level of energetic vibration.

Breathing

Proper breathing is essential when practicing a mudra. There are basically two types of breathing:

In *Long Deep Breathing*, you take your time inhaling and exhaling slowly and completely, through the nose.

When you inhale, relax the abdomen and expand the chest.

When exhaling, deflate the chest and pull in the stomach to help expel the air. This technique of breathing will help you relax, calm down, and be more patient.

In *THE SHORT BREATH OF FIRE*, inhale and exhale through the nose at a much faster pace. Focus on your navel point, expanding for inhalation and contracting on exhalation. Both parts are equal in time and can be quite rapid: two to three breaths per second.

This technique has a more invigorating effect.

Both techniques are very cleansing and healing.

During your mudra practice, it is best to use Long Deep Breathing except where noted.

Concentration

While practicing any mudra it is important to concentrate on the energy center of your Third Eye, which is between your eyebrows. Your Third Eye is the point of your body-mind that connects most easily to the higher sources of energy within you and around you.

As you practice meditation and mudra, if your mind wanders, gently bring your attention back to your breath and your mudra. Breathe in and out. You will experience a very powerful effect, a heightening of energy, throughout your entire body. Mudra practice affects each individual differently at different times. Sometimes you may feel a slight tingling sensation in your hands and arms; at other times, you may experience a sudden rush of energy through your spine. Allow yourself to feel and notice whatever comes up for you. Concentrating on the different feelings, allowing them to be there, will magnify the healing benefits to your body, mind, and spirit.

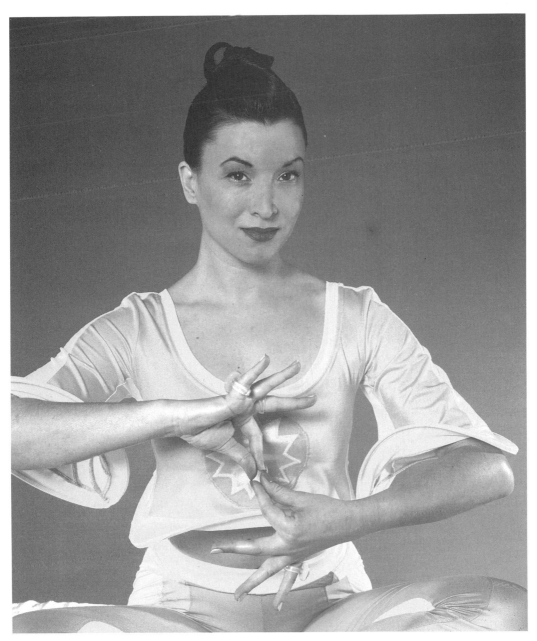

Mudra of the Wheel of Life—Yin and Yang.
Your Third Eye center is the point between the eyebrows.
By focusing your mind's attention on this energy center of intuition,
you can practice visualization and receive guidance and visions.
It is your window to infinite possibilities.

Eye Movements

The eyes are an important element in the practice of mudra. How you use them will increase your concentration.

You can keep them half open and gently direct them to look over the tip of your nose. Do not cross your eyes to do this. Just look down and slightly in so that you perceive the end of your nose. This is a very beneficial exercise for your eyesight.

Another practice is to close your eyelids and gently aim your eyes upward toward the area of the Third Eye.

If you need to keep your eyes open as you meditate, look into the middle distance and relax the eyelids.

Most important, the eye focus should always be done *gently*. Never force your eyes into a painful or uncomfortable position.

Visualization

We all know how to daydream. Actually, daydreaming is a form of visualization. In your mind you can create a picture, world, or dream in which you desire to live. Visualizing where you want to be and how you want to live and manifest your energy is the first step toward making your dream a reality. Mudra practice can help you actualize your dreams. The power of your mind is limitless. Live it, breathe it, and you will make it a reality.

For example: While practicing a mudra for anti-aging, visualize in your mind a healthy, youthful glow around your face. See yourself and your face vibrant and recharged. By adding the power of your mind to your daily practice of mudra and visualization, you will change and improve your outlook, your energy, and your entire life.

As another example, when practicing the mudra for insight, see yourself as having reached a happy solution for a problem you've been trying to resolve. Visualize how you would feel if your concern were over. From this visualization will emerge a positive approach to creating a good outcome.

Positive Affirmations and Prayer

When you meditate, your mind becomes fine-tuned to your body's needs and you gain in healing capacity. It is important before you meditate to make a positive affirmation for yourself. You can also affirm positive energy for another person, just as you would in a prayer.

Example: When practicing the mudra for dieting it is beneficial to affirm: "I am eating only healthful food. I am healthy, trim, and full. I am sticking to my diet." This simple affirmation will have a positive effect on you. When meditating or praying for someone else, it is helpful to see them surrounded by white or violet light and affirm: "My friend is healthy, happy, full of life, and smiling."

Your affirmation should always be formed in the present tense. "I am calm," not "I will be or want to be calm." Or, "I see the solution in my meditation." This positive statement creates powerful energy vibrations. Your energy is sent out into the universe and manifests your desires and intentions, enabling you to accomplish your goals successfully, honorably, and compassionately. Prayer and affirmations are especially powerful during the practice of mudra when your mind is calm and your concentration is magnified.

Mantra

While you may prefer to practice your mudra and meditation using your affirmation, you may also want to try using a mantra. Mantras are ancient Sanskrit healing words that have a powerful effect on your entire being when chanted repeatedly during meditation or mudra practice. The hard palate in your mouth has fifty-eight energy points that connect to your entire body. Stimulating these points with sound vibrations affects your mental and physical energy. Certain sounds that stimulate these points have a very healing quality. When you repeat aloud or whisper these ancient mantras or scientific healing-sound combinations, the meridians on your hard palate are activated in a specific order that repatterns the energy of your whole system.

There are three basic mantras that you will find in this book in different combinations:

EK ONG KAR
(One Creator, God Is One)

SA TA NA MA
(Infinity, Birth, Death, Rebirth)

HAR HARE HAREE
WAHE GURU
(Hah-rah; hah-ray; hah-ree; wa-hay; guh-roo)
(God Is the Creator of Supreme Power and Wisdom)

Not every mudra practice requires a mantra. All mudras can be practiced in silence to the rhythm of your breathing. You can use the mantras when you are struggling with a restless mind, since focusing on the words will help center you. Follow your intuition during the mudra practice and if you are drawn to chanting the mantras, try them when you feel it is right. You will experience profound peace, joy, and passion. Your soul will sing with the universe.

The Mantra Pronunciation Guide

A like the *a* in about
AA like the *a* in want
AY like the *ay* in say
AI like the *a* in sand
I like the *i* in bit
U like the *u* in put
OO like the *oo* in good
O like the *o* in no
E like the *ay* in say
EE like the *e* in meet
AAU like the *ow* in now

SAT rhymes with "what"
NAM rhymes with "mom"
WAHE—sounds like wa-hay
GU—sounds like "put."
Emphasize the "ch" at the end of every "such."
Pronounce the consonant *v* softly.
Roll the *rs* slightly.

When chanting a mantra like "Haree Har Haree Har," make sure you do not move your lips, and pronounce it with the tongue only.

The Hands

Both hands and all ten fingers have individual, distinct meanings. Each corresponds to the energy of a different body part and to the energy of our solar system. The right hand is influenced by the Sun and represents the male side of one's nature. The left hand is ruled by the Moon and represents the female aspect of one's nature.

The right hand is the receiver, while the left is the giver of positive powers. These meanings are also reflected in the hand positions of mudras. Each finger is associated with a special ability, tendency, or characteristic and how it affects your life.

The *Thumb* symbolizes God. When the rest of your fingers connect to the thumb you symbolically bow to God. The Thumb is associated with the planet Mars and represents willpower, logic, love, and ego. The angle it makes with the rest of your hand when relaxed indicates your character. A distance between the thumb and index fingers of around ninety degrees indicates you are generous, kindhearted, and giving. A distance of about sixty degrees suggests a logical, rational character. A thirty-degree space indicates a secretive, sensitive, and cautious person.

A long, strong thumb reveals a strong personality, willpower, and the ability to change your destiny.

The *Index* finger is influenced by the planet Jupiter and represents your knowledge, wisdom, sense of power, and self-confidence.

The *Middle* finger is the indicator of the planet Saturn and relates to patience and emotional control. Therefore, it has a balancing effect on your life.

The *Ring* finger connects with the Sun and represents vitality, life energy, and your health. It corresponds to your sense of family and matters of the heart.

The *Little* finger is the indicator for the planet Mercury, which rules your ability to communicate, be creative, appreciate beauty, and achieve inner calm.

The tips of fingers can reveal qualities of different natures. An oval fingertip can signify an impulsive person who needs motivation. A pointy fingertip is common for an independent, active person, and a square fingertip shows a logical and practical person.

The Chakras

Within our body, we have seven major nerve and energy centers that are located along the spine. The first is at the base of the spine, the seventh at the top of the head. These centers are called *Chakras*.

Their energy is always spinning clockwise within our bodies and influences—and is influenced by—our emotional, spiritual, and physical health.

In order to feel balanced and in harmony within ourselves and our environment, it is important that we know about these centers and their functions.

First Chakra

Represents: Survival, food, shelter, courage, will, foundation

Location: Base of the spine

Gland: Gonads

Color: Red

Second Chakra

Represents: Sex, creativity, procreation, family, inspiration

Location: Sex organs

Gland: Adrenal

Color: Orange

Third Chakra

Represents: Ego, emotional center, the intellect, the mind

Location: Solar plexus

Gland: Pancreas

Color: Yellow

Fourth Chakra

Represents: Unconditional true love, devotion, faith, compassion

Location: Heart region

Gland: Thymus

Color: Green

Fifth Chakra

Represents: Voice, truth, communication, higher knowledge

Location: Throat

Gland: Thyroid

Color: Blue

Sixth Chakra

Represents: Third Eye, vision, intuition

Location: Third Eye

Gland: Pineal

Color: Indigo

Seventh Chakra

Represents: Universal God consciousness, the heavens, unity, humility

Location: Top of the head, crown

Gland: Pituitary

Color: Violet

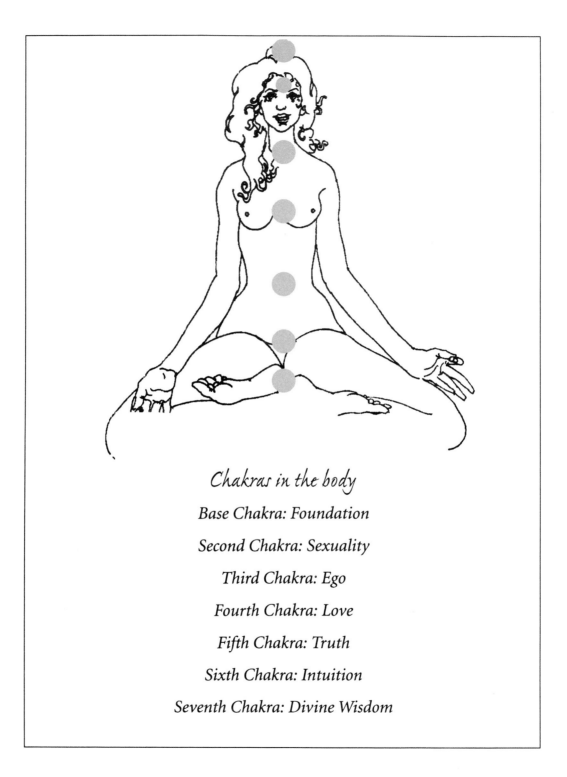

Chakras in the body

Base Chakra: Foundation

Second Chakra: Sexuality

Third Chakra: Ego

Fourth Chakra: Love

Fifth Chakra: Truth

Sixth Chakra: Intuition

Seventh Chakra: Divine Wisdom

Mudras are a powerful tool for energizing and balancing each Chakra, activating the electric current in our body, and releasing the limitless powers from within. *Example:* When practicing the mudra of divine worship (see frontispiece), you can visualize healing Chakra colors surrounding, filling, and energizing your body, starting with the First Chakra and continuing up to your head, the Crown Chakra.

Electric Currents

Besides the seven Chakras within our body, there are seventy-two thousand electric energy currents or channels called *Nadis* (pronounced "*nah*-dees"). They run from all different body points, from the tips of the toes to the top of the head. The Nadis also affect your entire system. Keeping these energy currents activated and full of powerful flowing energy is essential to your well-being. Each mudra redirects, activates, and empowers the energy flowing through those channels, and stimulates the brain centers, nerves, and organs, with benefits to your entire neuromuscular, physical, and glandular system.

Healing Colors

Using the healing power of colors can also enhance your mudra practice. The rainbow colors of Chakras heal and reenergize corresponding body parts. You can surround yourself with appropriate colors whenever you meditate or visualize the colors as you practice mudras.

For instance, when practicing the mudra for powerful insight, you can visualize yourself surrounded by white or violet light. This will enhance your intuitive capacity. Wearing a certain color will also influence your entire outlook on life.

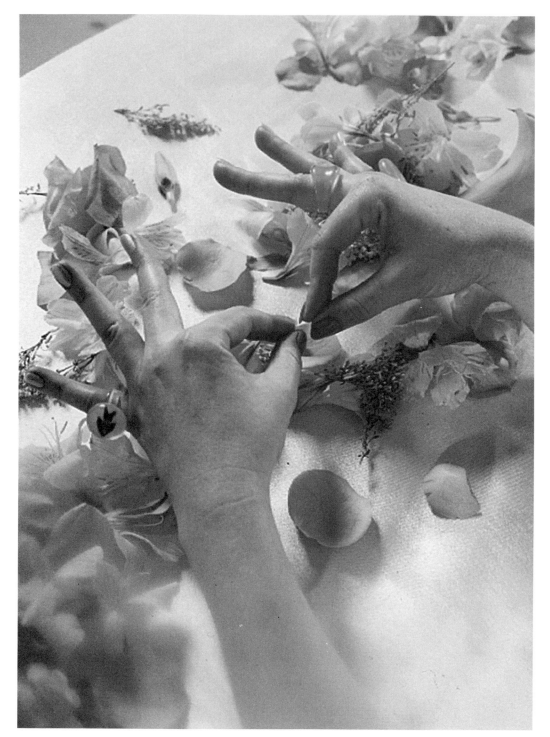

Mudra of yin—feminine power.

Examples:

Red will positively affect your vitality, ground you, and connect you to the earth.

Orange will empower your sexuality, creativity, and relationships.

Yellow makes you feel energized and full of fire.

Green is good for the days when you need to heal your heart and feel love.

Blue has a calming, peaceful effect on your aura or the energy field surrounding your body, and will help you see and speak the truth.

Indigo will enhance your intuition and sixth sense.

Violet is a great centering and calming color that will help you connect with the universal healing powers.

Black will help you communicate as a leader.

White will make you feel cleansed and pure, and it will help clear you of any negative feelings or depression.

Reflect on the messages your body sends you every morning, and see what color you feel most drawn to and comfortable wearing on different days.

The Aura

Our aura or energy body is made of electromagnetic energy vibrations that include color, light, sound, heat, and emotions. It surrounds us as a glow that is usually invisible. With practice and concentration, however, you can learn to see auras. The mudra for feeling the energy body is particularly effective in helping you to discern auras. When our invisible magnetic force is very vibrant, it signifies good health, personal power, and a healing capacity.

Useful Mudra Tips

Some mudras may seem at first to be very similar to each other. Yet each is, in practice, quite different: Every detail in the posture of your hands and fingers is important and significant. When you pay close attention to your practice of mudras, you will feel the difference. As we discussed, every fingertip is connected to a different body center and energy current. Concentrate on the mudra as you practice, and notice the different feeling and effect that each brings you. You can practice one specific mudra at a time or combine a few in one sitting. Listen to your body.

Example: If you are stressed out and need to concentrate, practice the mudra for preventing stress. After three minutes, go on to the mudra for concentration. As you try different combinations, your body-mind's logic and intuition will guide you. That is the beauty of the mudras—you can practice them anyplace, anytime, in whatever order you desire. This ancient science of the mudra is complex in benefits, yet simple in practice.

Now that you have some background about the power and history of mudras, and some rudiments of meditation practice, you're ready to begin trying some mudras and applying their energy to your life. In the next sections, you will find mudras for your soul, mudras for healing physical conditions, and mudras for easing troublesome states of mind, among others. Every one of these fifty-two traditional mudras can be a spiritual tool for you and help you in your own process of self-discovery and creative problem solving. I hope that they will enable you to find more insight, pleasure, and power on your life journey.

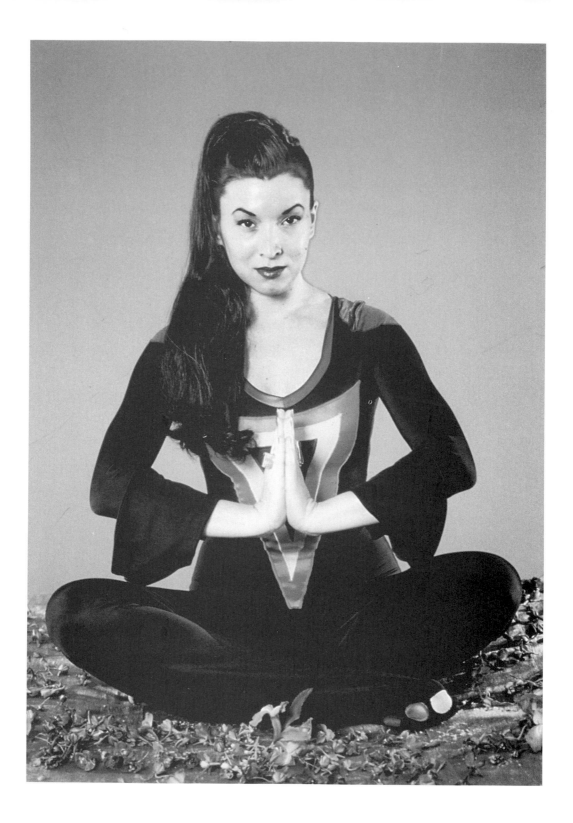

Part 1

Soul

Your soul is immortal . . .
Worship it.

This chapter contains sixteen mudras that will help you trust and connect with the energy of divine love, power, and wisdom, which is the source and sustainer of all living beings. When you need guidance, love, and inner strength, you can nourish your soul with the practice of mudra. Once you have met your own needs, you can continue to build up your own energy so that you are empowered and connected to the universe, able to help others in need.

You may practice one mudra a day or several. These will help you feel filled with peace, joy, and the knowledge that you are deeply loved and protected by your creator.

After the practice, take a few moments in complete peace and silence to feel the effects. If you do your part, holding yourself open to the Divine, the rest will be done for you.

Mudra for Divine Worship

The essential goal of yoga is to become centered, calm, and at one with the Divine, God, or the Universal Intelligence. Being respectful of the Higher Power, relying on it and being in tune with the universe, are prerequisites for inner peace. When we realize we are all created equal, and all connected with the ultimate source of spiritual energy, we feel empowered and in harmony.

The Mudra for Divine Worship is the universal symbol for prayer and has been used worldwide by saints and sages of many cultures and spiritual traditions. It sometimes begins with a bow to show our humility before the Divine Power. Connecting the palms and all fingertips symbolizes the unity and oneness with the Divine and magnifies the healing energy within ourselves.

Chakra: All Chakras

Color: All colors

Mantra: EK ONG KAR
(One Creator, God Is One)
Repeat mentally with each breath.

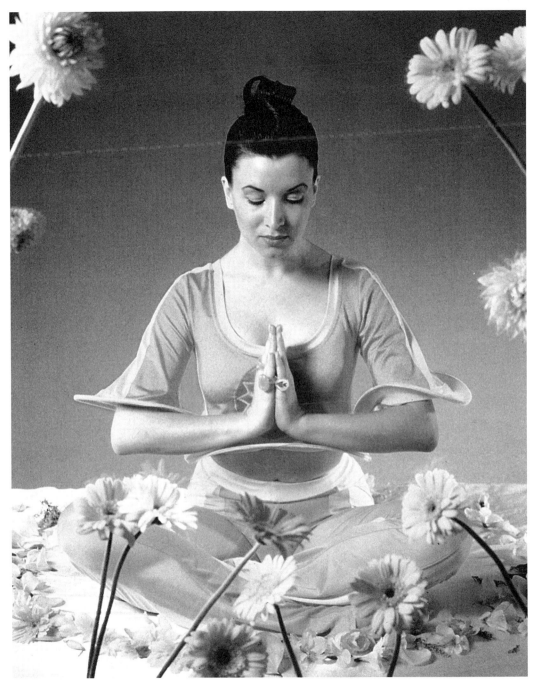

Sit in a comfortable position. Place your palms together in front of your chest. Concentrate on the Third Eye center. BREATH: LONG AND DEEP. *Relax your mind and continue for at least three minutes.*

Mudra for Happiness

Happiness is a state of mind that comes from within, just as true beauty emanates from our internal spiritual state. You can choose to make a conscious effort to greet each day and its events with a happy, positive outlook and to appreciate what you have. With regular practice of this mudra, you can be happy, look happy, and be a positive example to others. Make it a point to be happy today, tomorrow, and for the rest of your life.

The power of this mudra has a great effect
on your state of mind and
helps you feel joyful.

Chakra: Heart—4

Color: Green

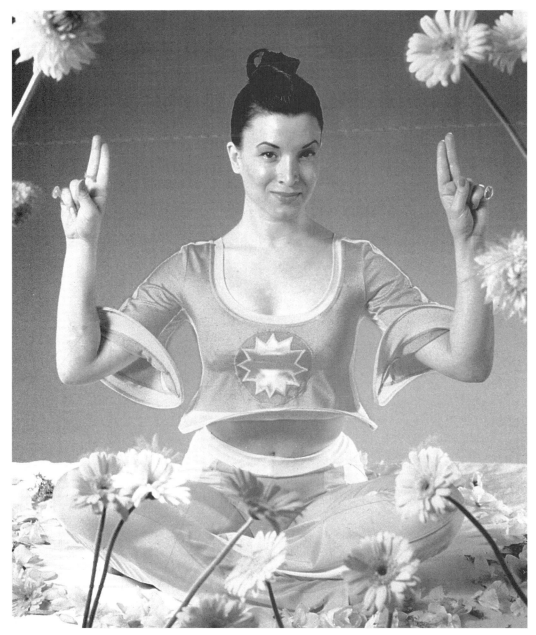

Sit comfortably with a straight spine. Curl the ring and small fingers and press them into your palms firmly but gently with the thumbs. Keep the first two fingers pointing straight up. Keep your spine straight and lift the elbows to the side and away from the body. BREATH: CONTROLLED, LONG AND DEEP, CONCENTRATING ON THE THIRD EYE AS YOU BREATHE.

Mudra for Love

Whether it is love for a child, parent, friend, lover, or any other living creature, love transforms us. It makes life worth living. Sharing our love with the world and teaching others about love is the spiritual mission at the base of every individual's life. Love yourself, humankind, and God, and you will achieve any goal.

This mudra activates the energy currents that stimulate the emotion of love.

Chakra: Heart—4

Color: Green

Mantra: SAT NAM WAHE GURU
(God Is Truth, His Is the Supreme Power and Wisdom)
Eight counts of breathing in, exhale to one count.
Mentally repeat the mantra twice when you inhale.

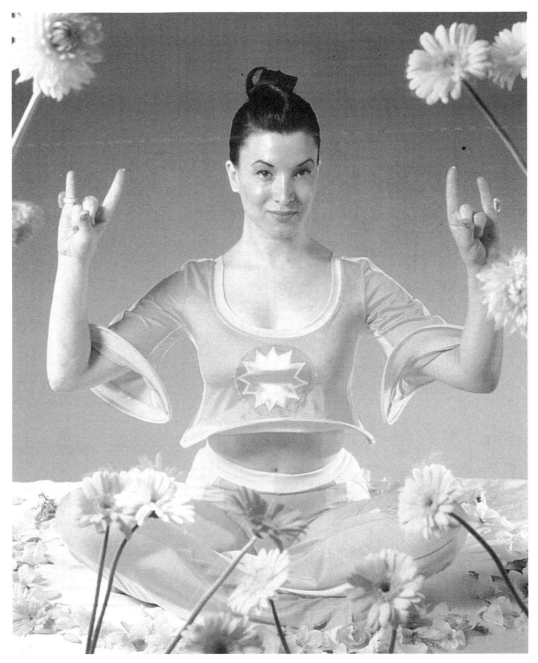

Sit with a straight spine. Curl the middle and ring fingers down into your palms while extending the thumbs and other fingers. Keep your elbows up, concentrate, and continue for a few minutes, feeling love and light around you. BREATH: *EIGHT COUNTS INHALATION, ONE STRONG EXHALATION.*

Mudra for Universal Energy and Eternity

We use only a small portion of our conscious mind every day. The practice of this mudra will stimulate your entire brain so that you can expand its capacity. By keeping energy flowing throughout your body and mind, and by learning how to recharge them every day, you stay in closer connection to the energy of life and the universe as a whole.

This mudra is beneficial for your whole system.
The hands are your channels to draw the life energy
into your body, mind, and soul.

Chakra: Base of the spine—1
Crown—7

Color: Red, violet

Mantra: HAR HARE HAREE WAHE GURU
(God the Creator of Supreme Power and Wisdom,
the Spiritual Teacher and Guide Through Darkness)
Repeat mentally with each breath.

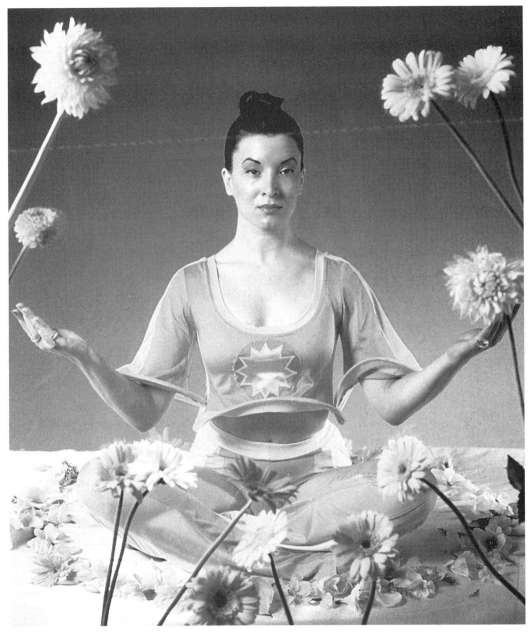

Sit with a straight spine. Bend your elbows, open your arms out to either side, and raise your hands up to heart level. Your arms and torso will form two V's. Keep palms facing up toward the sky with the fingers close together. Concentrate on your Third Eye and feel the flow of energy into your palms. Relax and feel a deep sense of peace. BREATH: LONG, DEEP, AND CONTROLLED.

Mudra for Trust

No relationship can exist for any length of time without trust. But first you must have faith and trust in yourself, your spirit, and in the greater wisdom of the universe. Do you trust yourself? Do you have faith in yourself? We are all connected to the ultimate creative force and Divine Spirit, which surround us and also lie within us. We are never alone and we are never forgotten. Self-trust and spiritual trust will help you attract people and relationships in which you have faith. The power of victory is always within you. It all starts with you.

This mudra will help you build trust, faith, and spiritual balance so that you can stand up to any challenge and see God in every aspect of your life.

Chakra: Crown—7

Color: Violet

Mantra: HAR HAR HAR WAHE GURU
(God's Creation, His Supreme Power and Wisdom)
Repeat mentally with each breath.

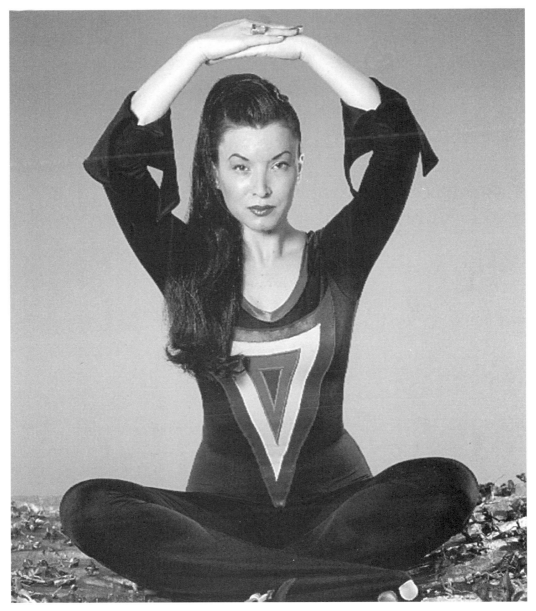

Sit with a straight back and make a circle with your arms arched up over your head, palms down. Women should put their right palm on top of the left. Men put the left palm on top of the right. Lightly press the thumb tips together, keep your back straight, and visualize a protective circle of energy all around you. BREATH: SHORT, FAST BREATH OF FIRE, FOCUSING ON THE NAVEL. *Hold the mudra and continue for a few minutes. Then relax and sit still.*

Mudra for Inner Integrity

We all encounter difficult situations that test our character. Even when we feel the impulse to react emotionally to a particular challenge, however, we must remember to act in accordance with the most intelligent, rational response. In maintaining our integrity we can save ourselves and our loved ones from a lot of sorrow, regret, and unnecessary pain.

When you are faced with such a challenge, take a few minutes to be by yourself, practice this powerful mudra, and notice your change of heart and mind.

This mudra will strengthen your ability to keep your presence of mind and inner integrity so that you can make correct choices and responses under stress.

Chakra: Throat—5
Third Eye—6

Color: Blue, indigo

Mantra: SAT NAM
(Truth Is God's Name, One in Spirit)
Repeat mentally with each breath.

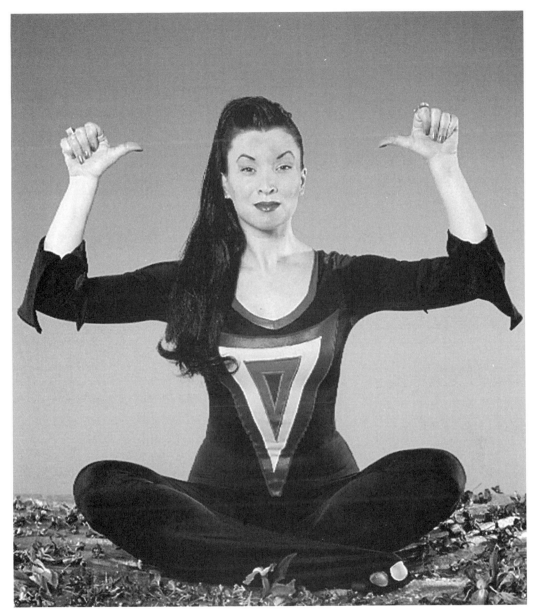

Sit with a straight spine, your upper arms raised parallel to the ground, your elbows bent so your forearms are perpendicular. Bring your hands to ear level, palms out. Curl your fingers inward so that they touch the palms. Extend your thumbs straight out and point them toward your temples. Practice for at least three minutes, then relax. BREATH: SHORT, FAST BREATH OF FIRE, FOCUSING ON THE NAVEL.

Mudra for Evoking Inner Strength

We all possess great reserves of inner power and wisdom. Within this innate understanding are all the answers and solutions to our problems. The practice of this mudra will help you tap into that well of inner strength. The mudra puts you in touch with the universal, everlasting force that lies within you.

As you hold the hand formations in front of your chest,
you are activating the power centers of the Third
and Fourth Chakras, which will give
you inner strength and courage.

Chakra: Solar plexus—3
Heart—4

Color: Yellow, green

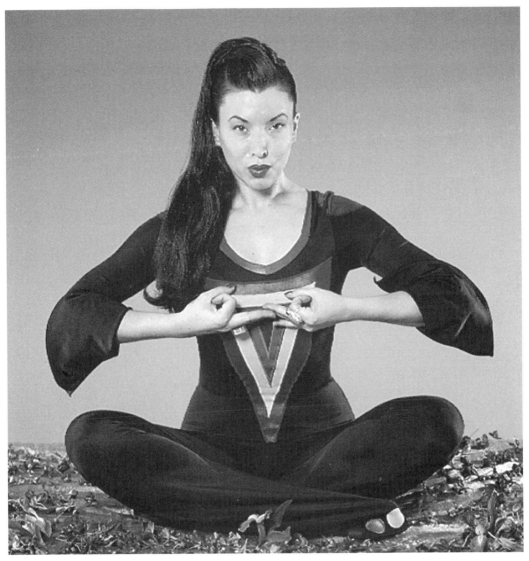

Sit with a straight spine. Curl your index fingers and curl your thumbs over them. Straighten the other three fingers. Your right hand is slightly under the left hand, your middle two finger pads touching the joints of the left hand. Place your hands in front of your chest, keeping your elbows up out to the sides so that your forearms and hands make lines parallel to the ground. BREATH: INHALE IN FOUR STROKES THROUGH THE NOSE, SHAPE YOUR LIPS INTO AN O, EXHALE WITH A WHISTLE. Continue for three minutes, then relax and feel the power within you.

Mudra for Wisdom

We can connect to our innate, divine wisdom by clearing our minds, concentrating, and practicing this ancient mudra. It will help you resolve any conflict you are facing by helping you see beyond your individual problems and into the bigger picture and higher meaning of any situation. This greater perspective will enable you to help yourself and others. This is a very powerful mudra, but it does require devoted practice. Do it every day for three weeks and you will be able to perceive more easily the answers to your questions and the purposes behind your life's challenges.

This mudra stimulates the mind nerve and clears your access to higher knowledge and wisdom.

Chakra: Third Eye—6
Color: Indigo

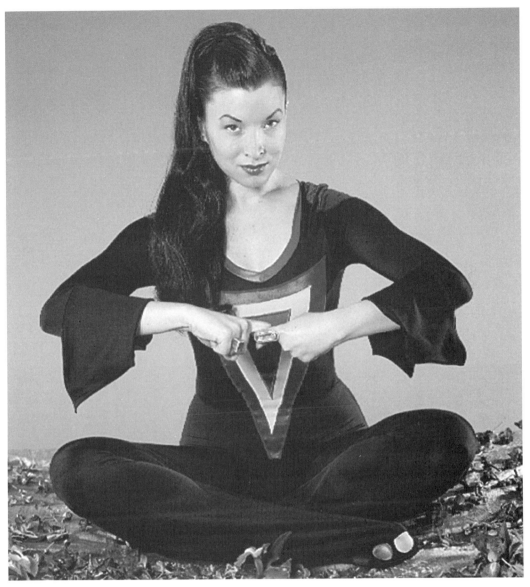

Sit with a straight back. Curl your thumbs into your palms and your last three fingers over them, leaving your index fingers extended. Keep your shoulders down and relaxed, but raise your elbows out to either side. Bring your curled hands in front of your chest and hook the index fingers together, right palm facing the ground, left palm facing your chest, forearms parallel to the floor. BREATH: LONG, DEEP, AND SLOW. *Hold the mudra for three to eleven minutes, relax, and sit still.*

Mudra for Gentleness

There are times when we are simply in a bad space at a bad time and feel harsh and unkind toward those closest to us. We may react unthinkingly, and while we may not mean what we say or do, our words or behavior can be very damaging. If we never learned or experienced calmness and gentleness as children, it may be difficult for us to be kind as adults. Gentleness is one of the highest soul qualities, however, and by cultivating it, we will be able to attract kind and loving people into our lives, and achieve a greater level of happiness and fulfillment.

This mudra will adjust the electromagnetic field of the brain and bring you calm and gentleness.

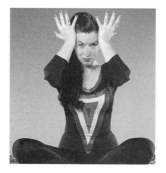 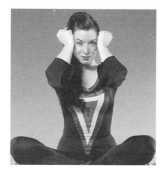

Chakra: Throat—5
Crown—7

Color: Blue, violet

Mantra: HARI ONG HARI ONG TAT SAT
(God in Action, the Ultimate Truth)
Repeat mentally with each breath.

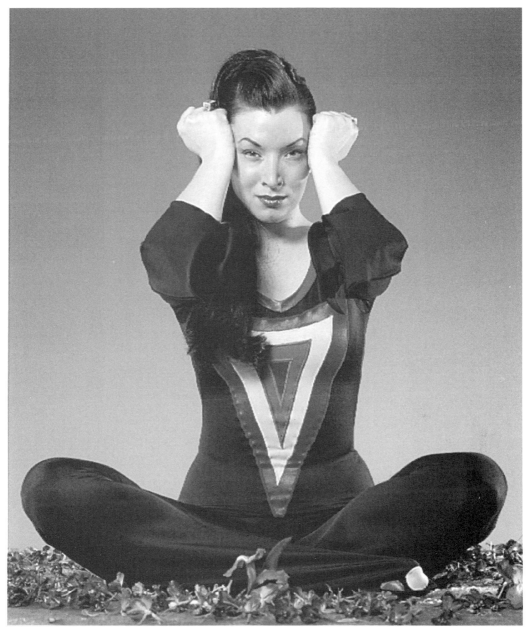

Sit with a straight back. Make fists and bring the outer (thumb) side of each fist to either side of your temples. Press the fists slightly against the temples and place the fingers apart. Close your eyes. Then make fists again, keeping the thumb sides pressing against the temples. BREATH: LONG, DEEP, AND SLOW. Practice for a few minutes, relax, and sit still.

Mudra for Developing Meditation

Some of us may struggle at the thought of sitting still for more than a few seconds. All of us have trouble sitting at different points of our life. Meditation is only a matter of discipline and practice. Learning how to still your mind and meditate even for a three-minute period is essential for your well-being. A short daily meditation will change your life for the better, and the sooner you start the sooner you will experience wonderful results on all levels and areas of your life.

This is a meditation for someone who cannot meditate.
It will bring one-pointedness and serenity to the most outrageous
or scattered mind. The mantra will help you focus with
the one universal force, "the heartbeat of life,"
that lies within us all.

Chakra: All Chakras

Color: All colors

Mantra: SAT NAM
(Truth Is God's Name, One in Spirit)
Repeat mentally with each beat of your pulse.

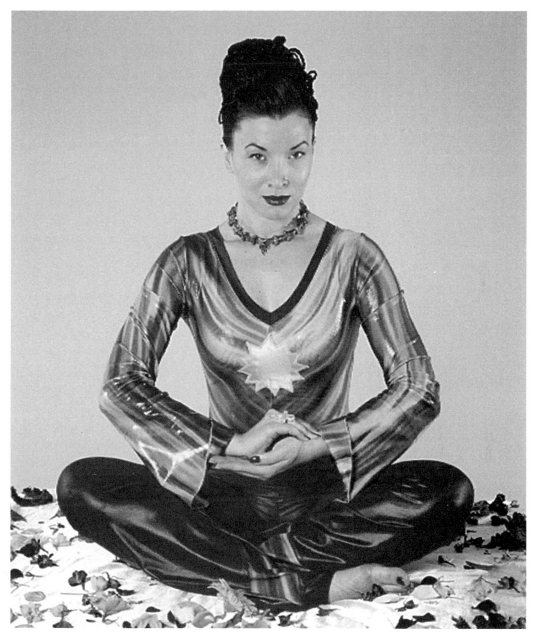

Sit with a straight back. With the four fingers of your right hand together in a straight line, feel the pulse on your left wrist. Press the fingers lightly so that you can feel the pulse in each fingertip. Palms are together. Close your eyes and concentrate on your Third Eye center. BREATH: LONG, DEEP, AND SLOW. Practice this mudra for three minutes daily for a week.

Mudra for Guidance

Spiritual knowledge and wisdom have been given to every soul in this world. The answers to all of your questions are within your heart and are available to you at all times, twenty-four hours a day, including weekends, free of charge, no waiting list, credit check, or reservations required. You have the VIP seat. All you have to do is calm down, get centered, relax, and use this mudra as the key to opening the door. Ask and you shall receive.

You receive energy and blessings into the palms of your hands.
Looking into them will send healing power to
your mind and help you find guidance.

Chakra: Crown

Color: Violet

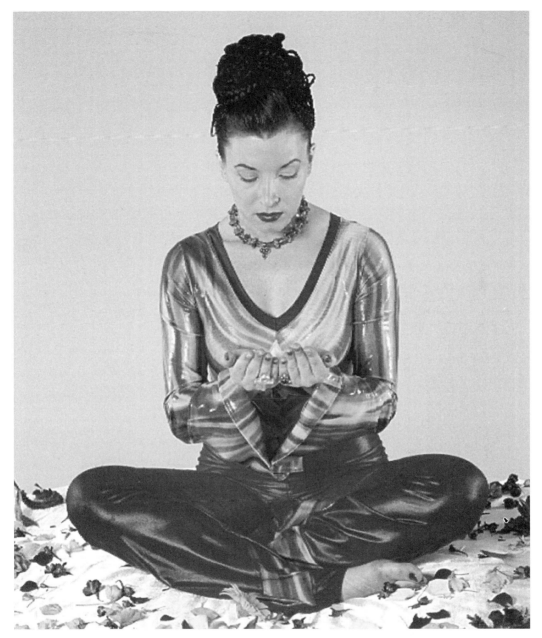

Sit with a straight spine. Put your hands together in front of your chest, little fingers pressed together to form a cup with the palms facing toward the sky. Leave just a small opening between the sides of the little fingers. Focus the eyes at the tip of the nose, toward the palms. BREATH: LONG, DEEP, AND SLOW INTO YOUR PALMS.

Mudra for
Help with a Grave Situation

Sorrow and sadness can come upon us suddenly, and it is important that we know how to keep ourselves together in spirit, mind, and body. Your heart is the center of emotion and love, and when an experience is particularly heartbreaking, you can actually feel physical pain in your chest and heart area. The healing power of your hands is used in this mudra to help you recharge, strengthen, and balance your heart and whole being.

This simple, ancient mudra will help you resolve any grave situation or conflict you are experiencing.

Chakra: Heart—4

Color: Green

Mantra: HUMEE HUM, BRAHAM HUM, BRAHAM HUM
(Calling upon Your Infinite Self)
Repeat mentally with each breath.

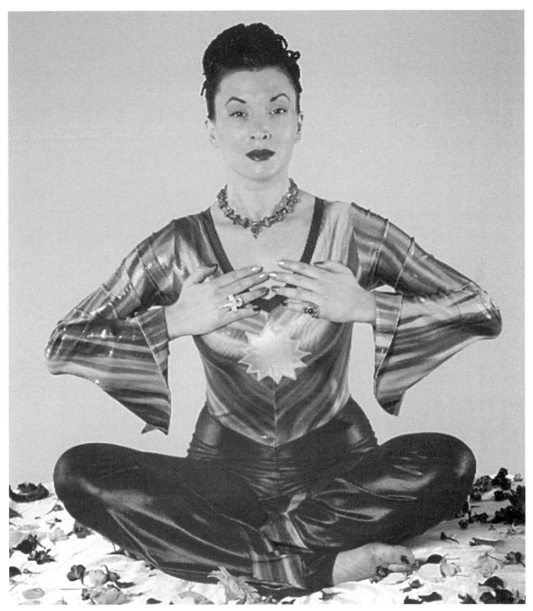

Sit with a straight spine. Place your palms on your upper chest, fingers point-ing toward one another, elbows out to either side. The hands are relaxed with the fingers extended. This is a comfortable position with very little pressure and no tension in the arms and hands. BREATH: LONG, DEEP, AND SLOW. Repeat a few times and notice calmness and peace surrounding you more each time.

Mudra for Powerful Insight

When you are unsure about what to do or how to remedy a problem, or you feel alone and confused, remember that you *can* find the answer within you. You just need to breathe deeply, calm down, and concentrate. With the help of this mudra, you will get the insight that you need. With regular practice, you will sharpen your intuition so that you may use it not only for yourself but also to help other people reach the same potential within themselves. We all possess the tools we need inside our souls.

This mudra coordinates both areas of the brain and stimulates the insight centers.

Chakra: Third Eye—6

Color: Indigo

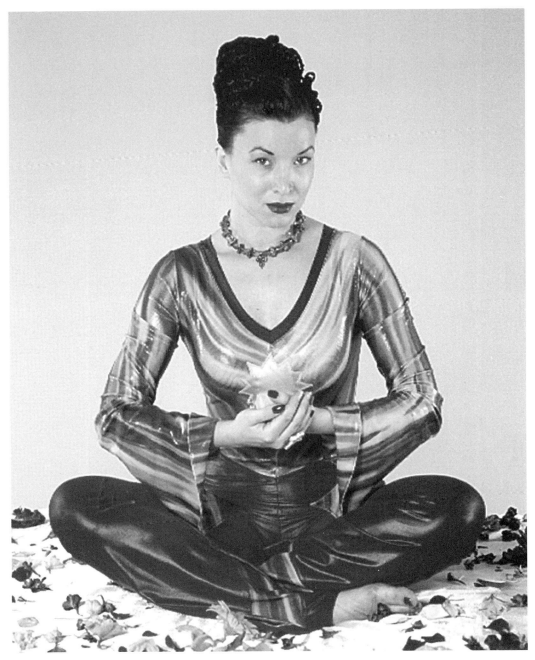

Sit with a straight spine, elbows out to either side. Raise your hands until they meet above the navel. The back of the left hand rests in the right palm and the thumbs are crossed, left over right. Concentrate on your Third Eye center. BREATH: LONG, DEEP, AND SLOW.

Mudra for Contentment

We all experience unhappy moments, but sometimes we carry them with us longer than necessary. Living in the past affects your present and your future, so it is important for you to get to a place of serenity and contentment from which to view your life. A few minutes of this mudra will give you immediate results. A daily practice will transform your life.

This mudra makes you feel cozy and content. The contact points between fingertips will redirect and balance your body energy and reinforce your inner ability to be in touch with your higher self.

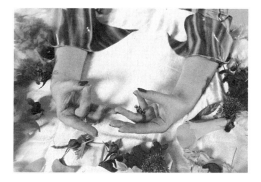

Chakra: Solar plexus—3

Color: Yellow

Mantra: SARE SA SA SARE
SA SA SARE HARE HAR
(God Is Infinite in His Creativity)
Repeat mentally with each breath.

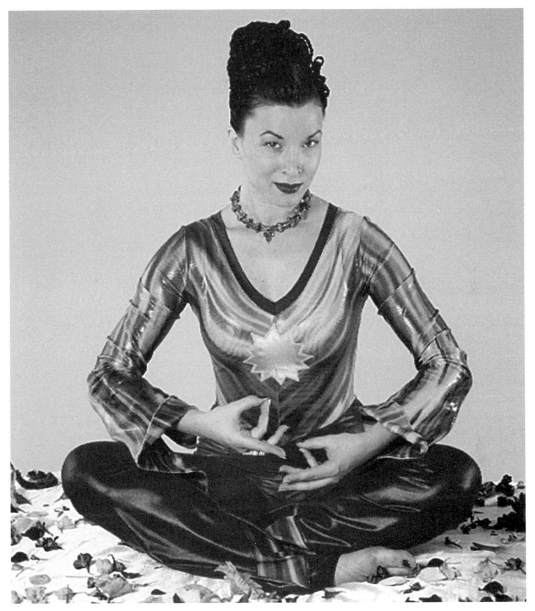

Sit with a straight spine. Make a circle with the thumb and middle finger of the right hand and the thumb and little finger of the left hand. Relax the other fingers. Hold the hands a few inches apart in front of your navel area. Men should make the same positions with the opposite hands. BREATH: LONG, DEEP, AND SLOW. Meditate for a few minutes, then make fists with both hands and relax.

Mudra for Prosperity

Physical, emotional, and material prosperity is your birthright. How do you achieve it? First, have a clear goal and intention. See yourself successfully achieving and living your dream. Then, with this mudra, you rid yourself of any mental and emotional energy blockage in your past that stands in your way. Next, you must make a practical, realistic plan of action.

Practice this mudra for eleven minutes every day for four weeks and see what happens. You should see your path clear and efforts rewarded.

You receive healing power into your palms with the motions of these hand positions. When you do this mudra with the chant "Har," you must and will manifest prosperity.

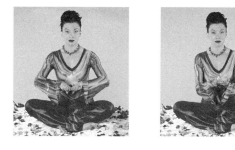

Chakra: Base of the spine—1
Reproductive organs—2
Solar plexus—3

Color: Red, orange, yellow

Mantra: HAR HAR
(God, God)
Repeat loudly with each exhalation, focus your energy on the navel.

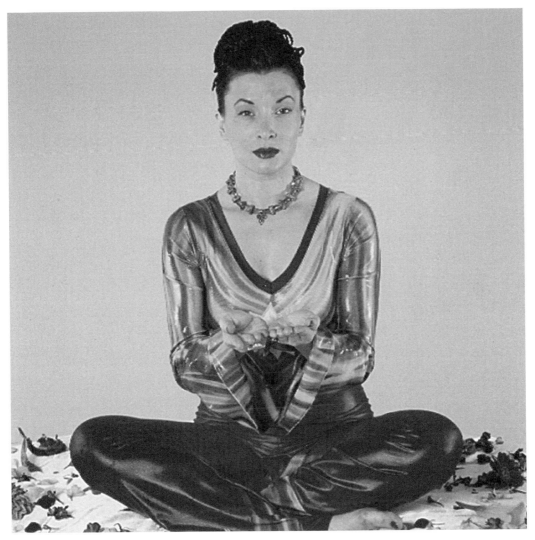

Sit with a straight spine and place the sides of your index fingers together, with thumbs hiding underneath the palms, palms facing the ground. Press the sides of the index fingers together firmly and hold for a second. Next, turn the hands over so the palms face the sky for one second, touching the hands together at the sides of the little fingers. Next, turn the palms toward the ground again, always keeping the sides of the hands touching. Each time you reverse the position of your hands, repeat the mantra "Har." Continue three to eleven minutes. BREATH: SHORT, FAST BREATH WITH EACH CHANGE OF HAND POSITION. BREATHE FROM THE NAVEL AND REPEAT THE MANTRA.

Mudra for Higher Consciousness

Higher consciousness is the ultimate goal of your life's journey. We all long to be able to maintain a state of calm centeredness in the midst of daily storms, when everyone else is fighting confusion. All the answers are within you, available to you at all times, but to gain access to this inner power requires proper practice and discipline. It is up to you. Whenever you search consciously, you will find the answer you need. You've known it all along.

This mudra will help you achieve higher consciousness, deeper intuition, and increased spiritual strength—all of which will give you understanding of the hidden purpose behind everyday events and challenges.

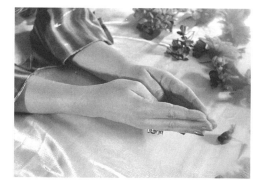

Chakra: Solar plexus—3
Crown—7

Color: Yellow, violet

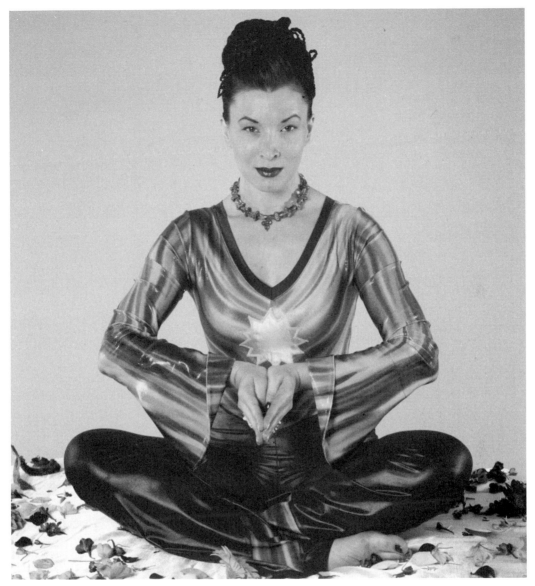

Sit with straight back. Put your palms together, extend your elbows out to either side, and lift your hands in front of your heart, fingers pointed away from you. Each thumb is on the fleshy mound below the little finger of the same hand. Put the palms together, with the right thumb snugly above the left thumb. The bottoms of the hands touch firmly. Hold the hands a few inches away from the body. BREATH: LONG, DEEP, AND SLOW. Repeat for a few minutes and build up your time. Relax and enjoy.

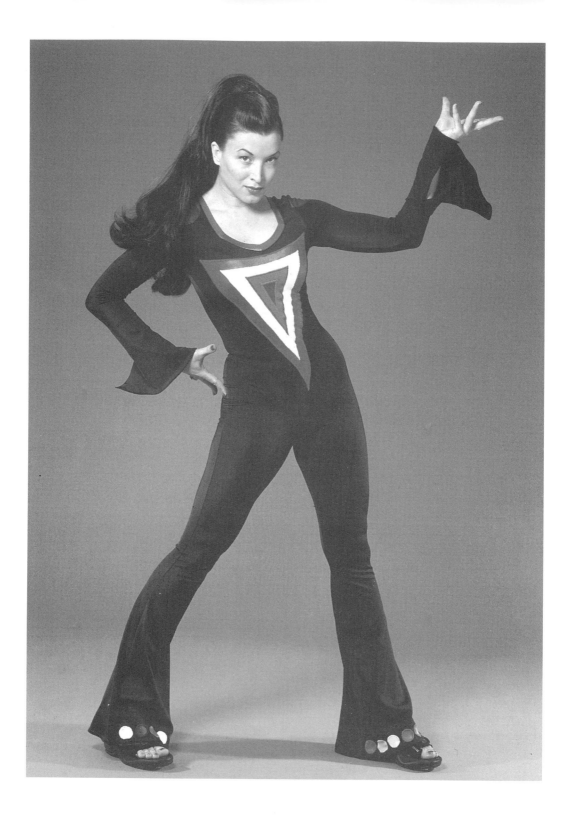

Part 2

Body

Your body is your temple . . .
Cherish it.

This chapter gives you fifteen mudras that will help you calm, heal, and reenergize your physical body. An amazing and sensitive creation, your body needs loving care, proper food, and exercise. Appreciate, love, respect, and celebrate your body. With daily practice of these mudras, you will learn to balance sexual energy, prevent aging and stress, conquer your addictions, physically relax, and recharge your body.

You can choose to practice only one mudra a day or as many as you wish until you feel energized, stress-free, and balanced. Be patient and practice self-love. See yourself with a healthy and vibrant body.

Mudra for Anti-aging

We all want to look young and healthy. A natural aging process is part of everybody's life, yet, no matter what your age, you can preserve and protect your body. Although a healthy lifestyle, with exercise and a proper diet, is essential, the most powerful ingredient of an anti-aging recipe is a proper state of mind. With this mudra, you can cleanse all the impurities in your system, reverse the aging process, and learn to enjoy the wisdom and experience that you gain with time.

This breathing technique and mudra will cleanse and brighten
your aura and regenerate your cells, which will give
you a radiant face and prevent aging.

Chakra: Base of the spine—1
Reproductive organs—2

Mantra: EK ONG KAR SA TA NA MA
(One Creator of Infinity, Birth, Death, and Rebirth)
Repeat mentally with each breath.

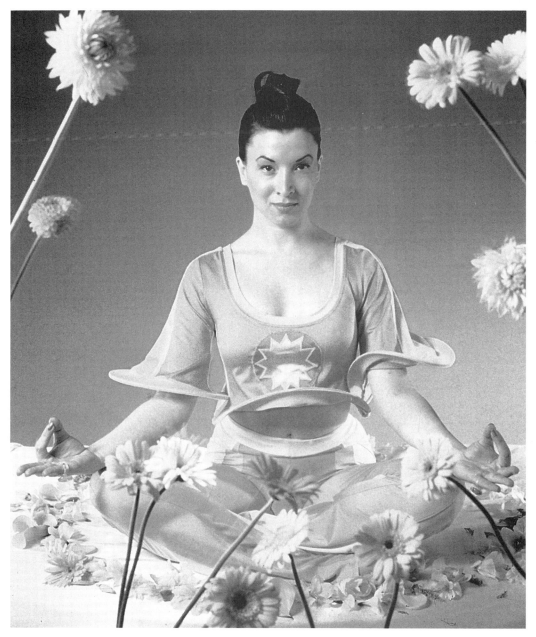

Sit with a straight back. Make circles with your thumbs and index fingers, and place the backs of your hands on your knees with palms up. Stretch the rest of your fingers out straight. BREATH: SHORT, FAST BREATH OF FIRE, FOCUSING ON THE NAVEL. THE BREATHING SHOULD BE SO POWERFUL THAT YOU "DANCE WITH THE NAVEL." *Practice for at least three minutes and relax.*

Mudra for Strong Nerves

You *can* learn to remain calm and centered in your everyday life, even in times of challenge and turmoil. You will instantly feel the power of this mudra as if you were connecting two currents of energy, yet its effects are soothing and calming and will keep your nerves strong.

This mudra will strengthen your nerves. By pressing the middle finger you are empowering emotional control, and the pressed little finger activates inner calm. Because female and male sides of the body correspond differently in men and women, the pose is reversed for men.

Chakra: Solar plexus—3
Heart—4

Color: Yellow, green

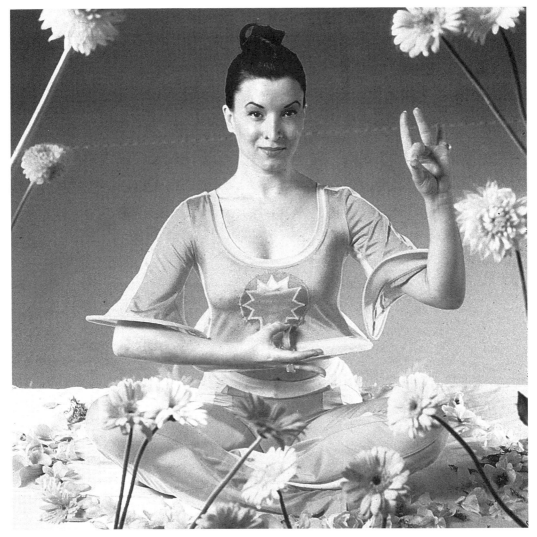

Sit with a straight spine and lift your left hand to ear level, palm facing out. Make a circle with the thumb and middle finger, and straighten the other fingers. The right hand is in front of the solar plexus, with the thumb and little finger touching, palms facing toward the sky. The rest of the fingers are straight. The position of the hands is reversed for men: *The right hand is held at ear level, with the thumb and ring finger held in a circle and the left hand in front of solar plexus with the thumb and little finger touching.* BREATH: INHALE IN FOUR COUNTS AND EXHALE IN ONE STRONG BREATH. *Continue for a few minutes.*

Mudra for Protecting Your Health

In addition to eating a proper diet, observing good hygiene, and getting regular exercise, you can preserve and protect your health by practicing this ancient and powerful mudra. Daily practice over many years will provide many benefits.

This mudra balances the distribution of red and white blood cells and defends your overall health.

Chakra: All Chakras

Color: All colors

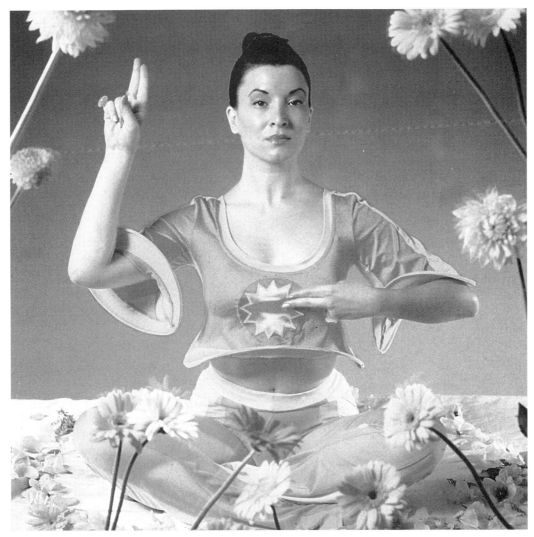

Sit with a straight back. Bend your right elbow and lift your hand up and out to the side as if taking an oath. Hold the first two fingers straight together and pointing up. Curl the other two fingers down into the palm and lock the thumb over them. Hold the left hand in the same mudra with the palm toward your chest, the two outstretched fingers touching the heart. Make the outstretched fingers as straight as possible to create a strong electromagnetic field around you. BREATH: TWENTY SECONDS INHALE, TWENTY SECONDS HOLD THE BREATH, TWENTY SECONDS EXHALE. Pull the navel in as much as possible. Continue for a few minutes and relax.

Mudra for Preventing Stress

We all experience stress in our lives. Many of us run from one activity to the next, taking care of too many things in a day without finding enough time to recover. It is very important for your body-mind to give it times in which it can slow down. Practicing this mudra for a few minutes, especially when you feel stressed out, can help. You will feel the results immediately and may find that you want to practice this mudra daily to build your energy for keeping stress-free.

This mudra enables the brain to maintain its equilibrium under stress and keeps the nerves strong.

Chakra: Solar plexus—3

Color: Yellow

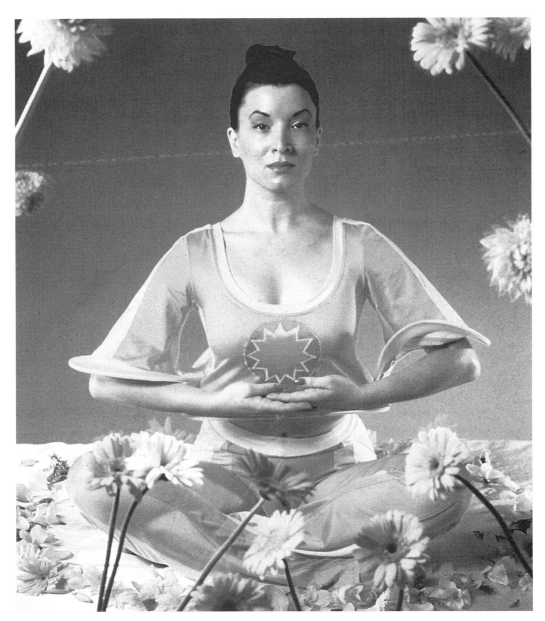

Sit straight. Relax your arms, bending your elbows to bring your forearms in front of you and parallel to the ground. Bring your hands, palms up, to meet in front of you, about one inch above the navel. Rest the back of the left hand in the palm of the right hand. Keep the fingers straight and together. BREATH: LONG, DEEP, AND SLOW. KEEP YOUR MIND FREE OF THOUGHTS. Repeat for three minutes and relax.

Mudra for
Healthy Breasts and Heart

Our bodies have great self-healing and disease-preventing capacities that work best when we use our consciousness to activate, utilize, and strengthen them. Mudras help the flow of electric currents within the body to keep you healthy and vibrating with healing energy.

In addition to any spiritual practice, every woman must perform regular breast self-examinations and stay in tune with her body, but this mudra will help the female system use energy to clean out the lymph glands in the upper chest, which preserves breast health.

The heart muscle is working constantly, so we must help it recharge and get some rest.

*This mudra will cleanse and recharge your chest area
with self-healing energy. Daily practice will keep the heart strong.*

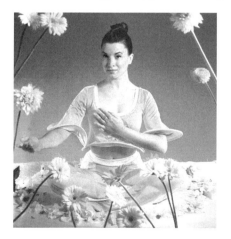 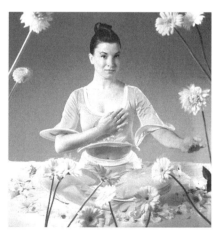

Chakra: Heart—4

Color: Green

72

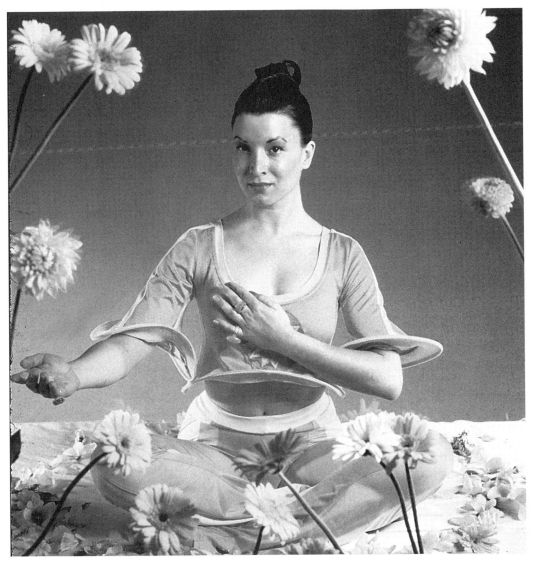

Sit calmly in a comfortable posture, back straight. Relax your arms at your sides with the palms facing forward. Then alternately bend each elbow so that the forearms come up toward the heart center as rapidly as possible. When your right hand is at your chest, the left hand is away from the body, and when the left hand is in front of your chest, the right hand is away from the body. Do not bend the wrists or hands and do not touch the chest. Continue at a rapid pace four times while you inhale, four times while you exhale, until you feel hot, then relax for a few minutes. BREATH: LONG, DEEP, AND SLOW.

Mudra for
Feeling Your Energy Body

The physical body is surrounded by an invisible energy body, or aura. With training, you can learn to perceive this vibrant halo that surrounds you. As you practice this mudra, breathe and concentrate, and you will begin to sense, see, and feel your energy passing between your palms. Regular practice will increase your ability.

*By directing the palms and their auric energy glow
toward each other, you magnify the energy field
and can therefore perceive it more easily.*

Chakra: Third Eye—6
Color: Indigo

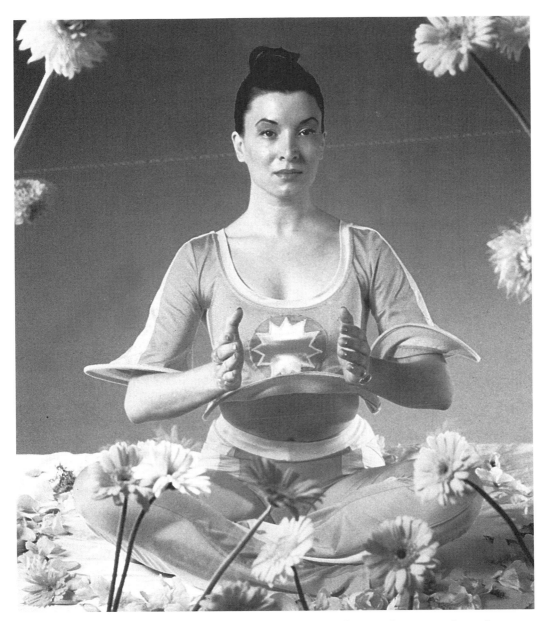

Sit with a straight spine. Bring your palms in front of you so that they are open and facing each other. The fingers are slightly apart and slightly cupped. The tips of the fingers are pointed away from you. Breathe long, deeply, and slowly. Keep the eye focus between the palms. As you breathe, feel the energy flow from one hand to the other. After a few minutes, you will begin to see the flow of energy. BREATH: LONG, DEEP, AND SLOW.

Mudra for Preventing Burnout

When you don't give yourself the proper rest that you need and deserve, you can endanger your mind-body health and drain your life energy. Whenever you feel so tired that it seems impossible to recover, this is the moment for gathering your last sparks of energy and practicing this mudra. Even if it is difficult to hold the mudra in the beginning, after three minutes you will feel rejuvenated and surprise yourself with the power that is within you.

The pressure of your fingers stimulates your electric currents and recharges them with vital energy.

Chakra: Base of the spine—1
Reproductive organs—2
Solar plexus—3

Color: Red, orange, yellow

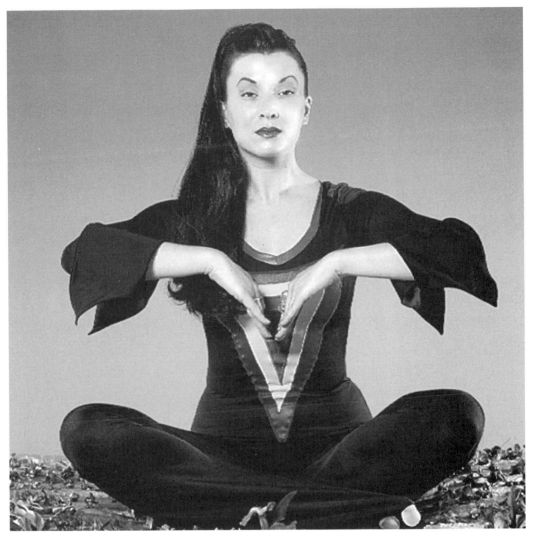

Sit with a straight back, bend your elbows, and raise your forearms up and in front of you, parallel to the ground, hands meeting at the level of the heart, palms facing the ground. Fold the thumbs in across the palms of each hand until the thumb tips rest at the bases of the ring fingers. Keep the four fingers straight and together. Face the backs of the hands toward each other and press only the fingertips together. Firmly press the fingertips and nails of each hand together, the upper hands not touching. Deeply inhale and completely exhale. BREATH: LONG, DEEP, AND SLOW. Repeat a few times and relax. Rest for a few minutes.

Mudra for
Healing After a Natural Disaster

Earthquakes, floods, tornadoes, and other natural disasters are unfortunately quite common. After such a traumatic upheaval, people feel disoriented, confused, vulnerable, and fearful. This mudra can have an immediate, powerful, positive effect and help you get through the aftermath of the crisis and realign your own energy with that of the earth.

This mudra will readjust the magnetic relationship of the two hemispheres of the brain, which will help you regain emotional balance.

Chakra: Base of the spine—1
Solar plexus—3
Third Eye—6

Color: Red, yellow, indigo

Mantra: HARI ONG TAT SAT
(God in Action, the Ultimate Truth)
Repeat mentally with each breath.

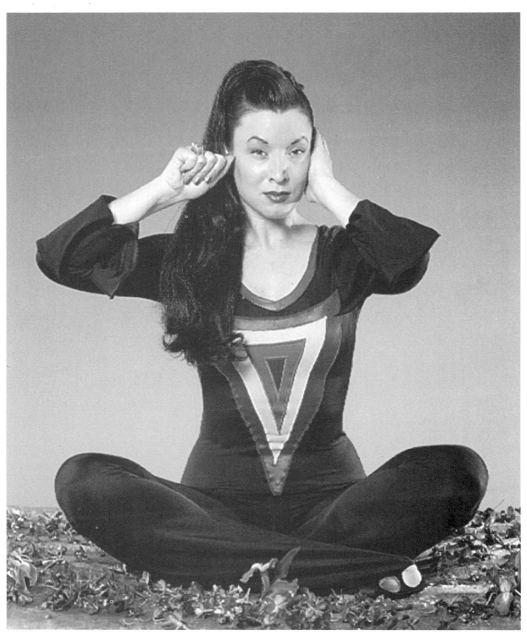

Sit up straight. Slightly cup your left hand and hold it over your left ear, keeping your left upper arm parallel to the ground. Make a fist with your right hand and extend your right arm straight out to your side, then bend your elbow so that your fist is by your ear, palm slightly away from you. BREATH: LONG, DEEP, AND SLOW. *Continue for a few minutes and relax.*

Mudra for Overcoming Addictions

Addictive habits are a very common problem. All addictions are connected to our desire to avoid accepting that we are individuals responsible for ourselves. Our addictions let us feel less alone but also keep us from facing the reality of certain problems or situations. We try to alter our troubling moods and upset feelings by using addictive substances or distract our attention from ourselves with addictive relationships.

To overcome an addiction, you must overcome the fear behind it. You need to realize at your deepest level that nothing is as bad as you fear. Distracting yourself with drugs, caffeine, alcohol, cigarettes, food, or bad relationships only worsens the problem. It also delays your achievement of your purpose in life.

You can overcome any addiction; you just have to set your mind to it. The regular practice of this mudra for three minutes, three times a day will help you overcome any addiction in thirty days. Set yourself free from the chains of addiction and begin this practice of self-love today.

This mudra works on physical addictions as well as emotional addictions and codependence. The pressure of your thumbs on your temples triggers a rhythmic reflex current into the central brain that balances the energies that cause addictions.

Chakra: Base of the spine—1
Reproductive organs—2
Solar plexus—3
Heart—4
Throat—5

Color: Red, orange, yellow, green, blue

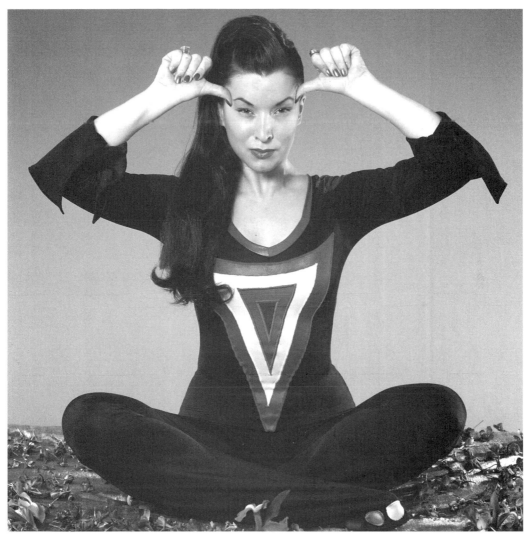

Sit with a straight spine. Make sure you are not slouching, especially in your lower back. Make fists with your hands and then extend the thumbs out. Press the thumbs on the temples where you feel a slight depression. Clench your teeth, lock the back molars, and keep your lips closed. Vibrate the jaw muscles by alternating the pressure on the molars. A muscle will move in rhythm under the thumbs. Feel it massage the thumbs as you continue to apply firm pressure with them. Concentrate on your Third Eye center as you do this. Continue for three to eleven minutes. Now relax your arms and place them at your sides, with the thumbs and index fingers forming a circle. Hold the pose and relax. BREATH: SHORT, FAST BREATH OF FIRE, FOCUSING ON THE NAVEL.

Mudra for Healing a Broken Heart

When you are in the middle of grief and heartbreak, it seems pretty impossible to escape the experience. Sadness seems overwhelming initially, but with time you can come to understand why you had to go through that pain. Whatever the larger reasons, while we are going through this painful experience, we can heal our heart faster with this beautiful mudra.

*This mudra is very relaxing and good for the nerves, and
it will calm and heal a broken heart.*

Chakra: Heart—4
Throat—5
Third Eye—6

Color: Green, blue, indigo

Mantra: HUMME HUM HUM BRAHAM
(Calling upon Your Infinite Self)
Repeat mentally with each breath.

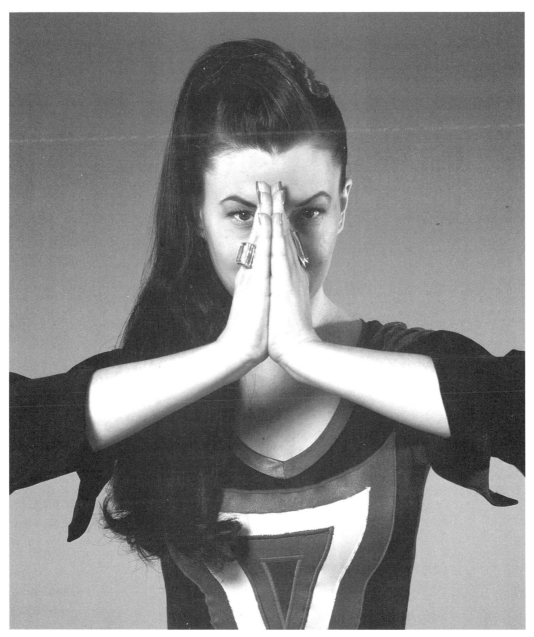

Sit with a straight back. Hold the palms lightly together, with the tips of the middle fingers at the level of the Third Eye center. The arms are horizontal, elbows out to the sides. Hold this mudra for at least three minutes. BREATH: LONG, DEEP, AND SLOW THROUGH THE PALMS OF YOUR HANDS, AS IF DRINK-ING WATER.

Mudra for Eliminating Fatigue

When the feelings of fatigue and exhaustion just overwhelm you, you can feel better with this simple mudra. Take a few moments to yourself, calm down, and breathe.

This meditation will bring healing, boost your energy, and enhance your intuition.

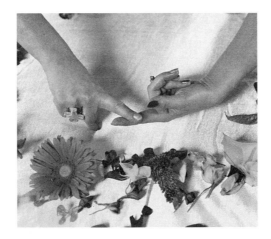

Chakra: Solar plexus—3

Heart—4

Color: Yellow, green

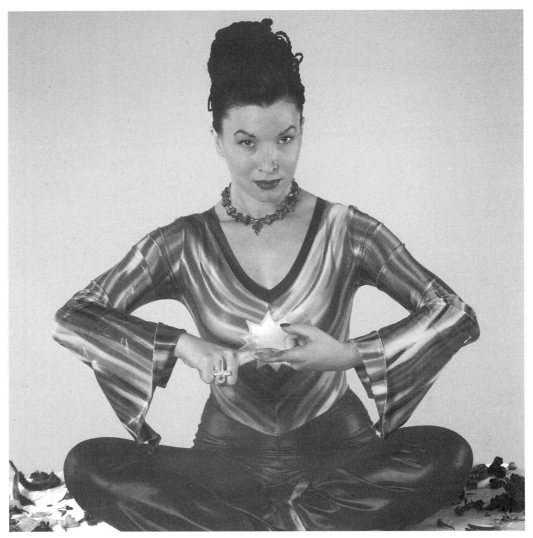

Sit straight. Elbows out to the sides, hold your hands level, in fists, at the solar plexus, except for the index fingers, which are straight. Hold the right palm down, left hand palm up. Put the right index finger on top of the left index finger. The fingers are crossing exactly in the middle of the second segment so that a special meridian contact takes place. BREATH: INHALE LONG, DEEP, AND SLOW BREATHS THROUGH THE NOSE AND EXHALE THROUGH THE PUCKERED MOUTH SLOWLY, WITH FORCE, DIRECTING THE BREATH AT THE TIPS OF THE INDEX FINGERS. Meditate on the sensation of your breath on your fingers and continue for a few minutes.

Mudra for Dieting

True beauty comes from the inside out. We each have a unique beauty, however, that is affected by what we eat. When we eat healthful food, we will have a healthful and vibrant appearance. If you crave junk food, this mudra will help you keep to your diet and curb your appetite, and it will still leave you feeling energized.

This mudra will build up your electromagnetic field and allow you to draw energy from the universe so that you can easily maintain your body with less food.

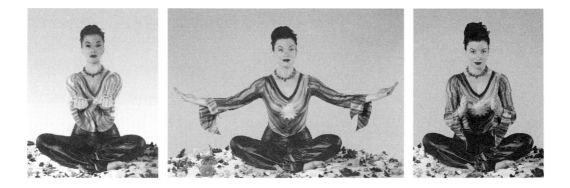

Chakra: Base of the spine—1
Solar plexus—3
Crown—7

Color: Red, yellow, violet

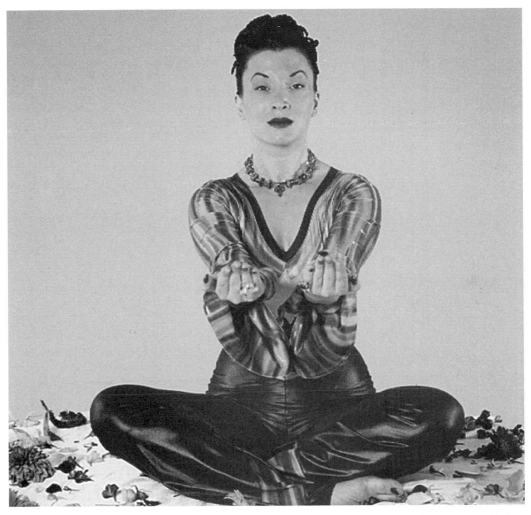

Sit with a straight spine and extend your arms out in front of you, parallel to the ground with palms facing up, hands slightly cupped. Very slowly move your arms back to your sides as far as possible, keeping them parallel to the ground with palms up. Then return your arms very slowly to their original position so that the sides of the palms almost touch in front of you. Repeat. Feel the energy coming through your Crown Chakra to your palms. As the palms come together, feel and resist the attraction. This maneuver builds up the energy in you. Continue for at least three minutes. As you end, relax your hands in front of your chest, with elbows bent and palms facing each other. Keep the palms three inches apart and visualize a ball of energy between them. Continue for a few minutes and relax. BREATH: LONG, DEEP, AND SLOW.

Mudra for Recharging

We all need to know how to recharge and rejuvenate our minds and bodies to keep up with personal and professional daily demands. You can practice this mudra anytime, and virtually anyplace. After just a few minutes you will feel a difference.

This mudra builds up energy throughout your system and gives you a greater capacity for dealing with life's challenges and tasks. The hands in this mudra activate and recharge the main energy channel in your spine, filling it with new vibrant force.

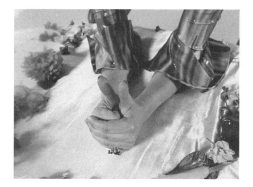

Chakra: Base of the spine—1
Reproductive organs—2
Crown—7

Color: Red, orange, violet

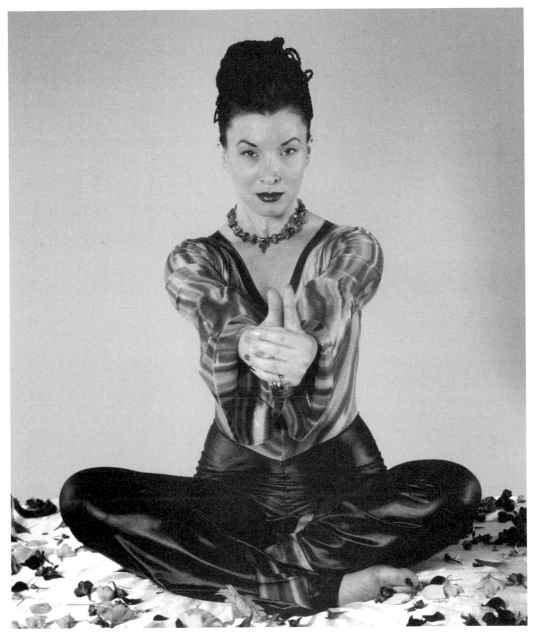

Sit with a straight spine and extend your arms straight out in front of you, parallel to the ground. Make a fist with your right hand. Wrap your left fingers around the fist, with the bases of the palms touching, thumbs close together and extended straight up. Focus your eyes on the thumbs. BREATH: CONTROLLED, LONG, DEEP, AND SLOW. Continue for a few minutes and relax.

Mudra for Balancing Sexual Energy

We are constantly bombarded with sexual stimulants, distractions, and exploitations in commercials and advertisements. These images and attitudes actually deplete our essential sexual energy and make our sexual relationships difficult. Yet sex can be a beautiful, giving, spiritual experience of two souls, which must be respected and cherished. During sex, a powerful exchange of two creative forces occurs that affects us for a long time, so it is most important that we keep our sexual energy balanced and nurtured. Negative past experiences can be healed and the ultimate sexual power and pleasure can be achieved when we consciously channel this energy.

This mudra balances and channels your sexual energy. It cleanses and recharges the glands that affect your entire sexual and reproductive system. For strength and confidence in your sexuality, the right thumb is on top of the left. For sensitivity and gentleness, the left thumb is crossed over the right thumb.

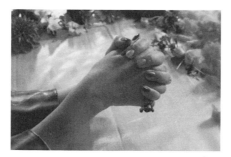

Chakra: Reproductive organs—2

Color: Orange

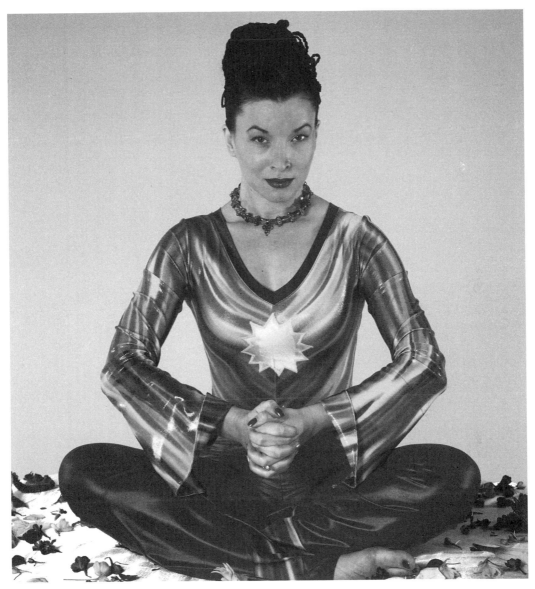

Sit with a straight spine, elbows slightly out to the sides. Clasp your hands together, interlocking your fingers. Leave the left little finger outside of the hand. By placing the right thumb on top of the left thumb we empower our masculine side, and when the left thumb is placed on top of the right thumb we recharge the feminine side of our nature. Press your hands together in this mudra, hold for three minutes, and relax. BREATH: INHALE AND EXHALE STRONGLY THROUGH YOUR NOSE.

Mudra for Longevity

With proper diet, exercise, and this ancient mudra technique, you can prolong your life. Your body rhythm is the determining factor for your longevity, and this mudra taps into the energy of that clock and fine-tunes it. With regular daily practice for three minutes, three times a day, you will enhance and prolong your life span.

This mudra works on the life nerve, which runs along your spinal cord and helps create a new body rhythm, increasing your longevity.

Chakra: Base of the spine—1
Crown—7

Color: Red, violet

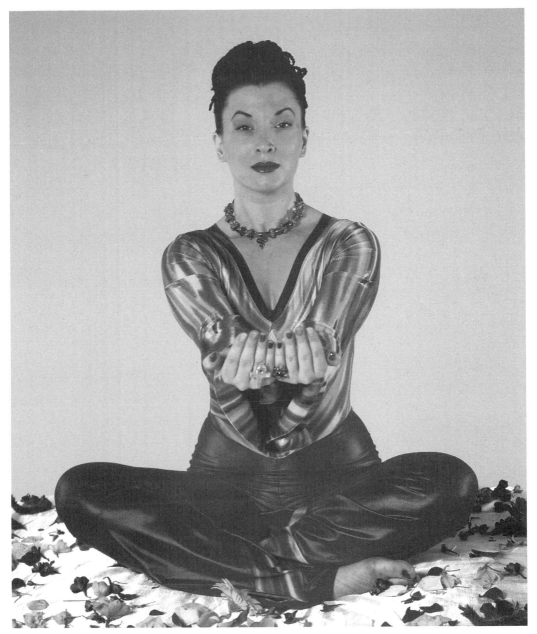

Sit with a straight spine and stretch your arms in front of you parallel to the ground with elbows straight. Palms are facing up toward the sky. Cup your hands together as if water were about to be poured into them. Hold for at least three minutes and relax. BREATH: SHORT, FAST BREATH OF FIRE, FOCUSING ON THE NAVEL.

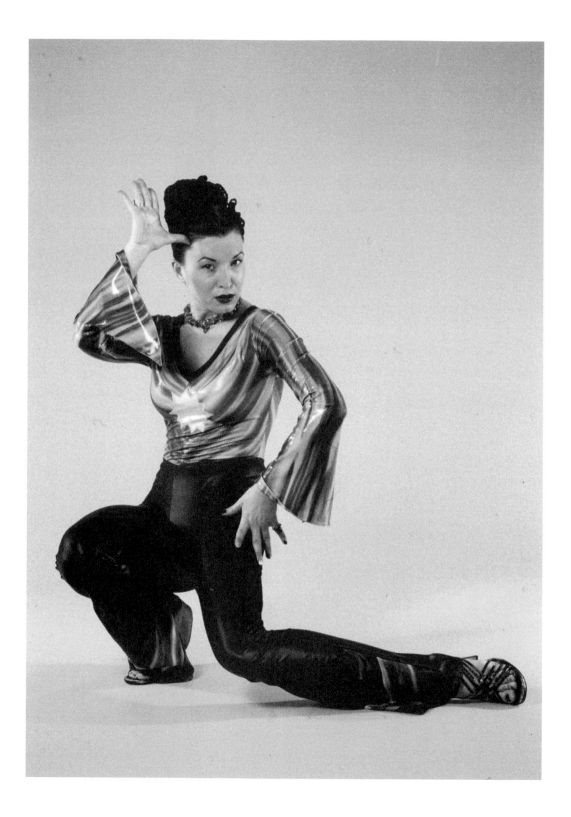

Part 3

Mind

Your mind has no limitations . . .
Expand it.

These twenty-one mudras for the mind are helpful with a variety of problems that you have created for yourself—in your mind. A confused state of mind is like a wild horse running. With discipline, you can rein in the energy of your wild thoughts and master your mind. When you teach your mind who is in charge, anything and everything becomes possible. Chase away your self-created ghosts of fear and insecurity and experience the immense power of your mind with these yoga practices.

You have been given a divine gift of free will. What you do with it, you alone decide. We create our own destiny, and with a sharp mind, you can define, correct, and change your destiny for the better.

You can practice one mudra a day or as many as you wish, until your fears and other mental obstacles disappear. As your mind clears, you will see how to use it to help yourself and others. When you act for the good of this world, you will never be alone.

Bedtime Mudra for a Good Morning

The way we feel in the morning affects our entire day. Waking up positive and rested, full of energy and inspiration, will help us live a happier, healthier, more fulfilled, and adventurous life.

This mudra must be done at bedtime to give you a positive frame of mind in the morning. As you practice it, visualize a white ball of light above your head. You will start the next day protected and surrounded by white light.

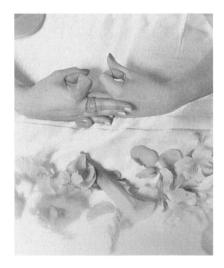

Chakra: All Chakras

Color: All colors

Mantra: HAR HARE WAHE, HAR HARE WAHE
(God Is the Creator of Supreme Power and Wisdom)
Repeat mentally, with six strokes of inhale and one long exhale.

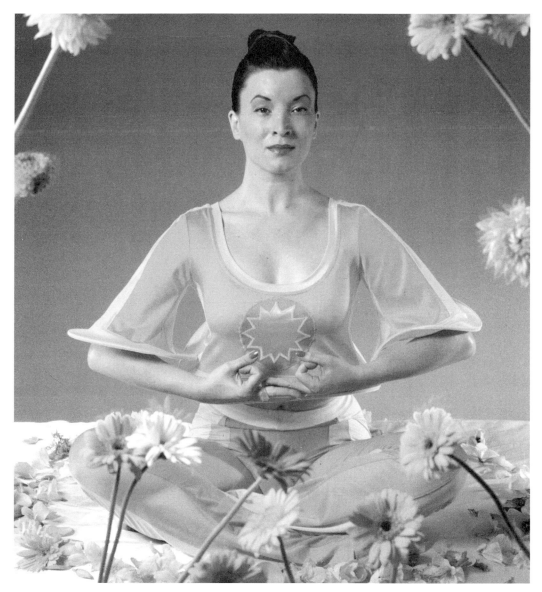

Sit with a straight spine, elbows extended to the sides, hands a few inches in front of the body, just above the navel. Your palms are facing up. Curl your thumbs around the index fingertips and extend the middle, ring, and little fingers so that they touch each other back to back. Keep your palms up, left hand on top of the right. BREATH: INHALE SIX SHORT BREATHS AS YOU MENTALLY REPEAT THE MANTRA AND EXHALE IN ONE STRONG BREATH. *Continue for three minutes and build up your time to eleven minutes.*

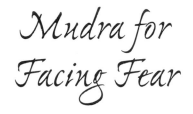

Mudra for Facing Fear

Fear prevents us from achieving our goals and dreams. Sometimes the energy you create by being afraid of certain things will actually attract those exact situations into your life. When we give fear too much power over us in our own mind, we may see "our worst fears come true." If this occurs, see it as an opportunity to deal with the fear and conquer it.

The right hand is symbolic of divine protection; the left hand symbolizes your receiving this gift. This mudra will help you diminish all feelings of fear. It is used in many cultures and is very powerful.

Chakra: Solar plexus—3
Crown—7

Color: Yellow, violet

Mantra: NIRBHAO NIRVAIR AKAAL MORT
(Fearless, Without Enemy, Immortal Personified God)
Repeat with each breath.

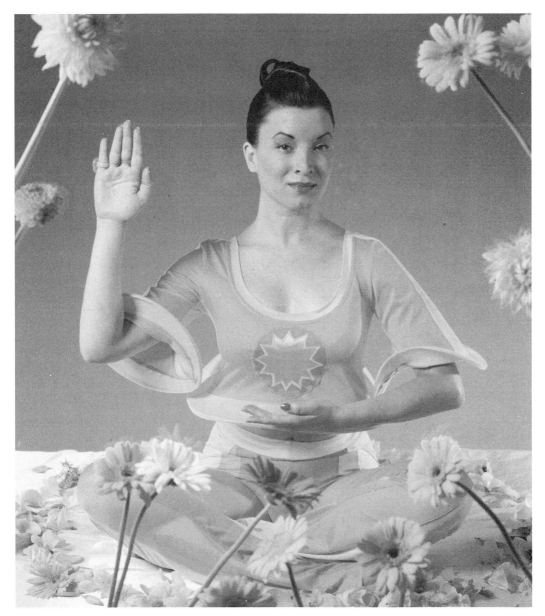

Sit with a straight spine, bend your left arm at the elbow, and hold your hand in front of your navel with the palm up. Lift your right arm and hold your hand in front of your right shoulder with the palm turned outward, fingers and thumb straight up. Concentrate on your Third Eye. BREATH: LONG, DEEP, AND SLOW. See yourself protected, inhale that positive feeling, and exhale the negative fear.

Mudra for Releasing Guilt

We all carry with us some feelings of guilt. Maybe somewhere in our past we behaved selfishly or angrily. Maybe we feel we don't really deserve to be happy, fortunate, or loved. Negative past experiences can be blocking us from moving forward in our lives with optimism and joy. Forgiving yourself is a necessary step for achieving a fulfilled, healthy, and happy life. The practice of this mudra is the first step to freeing your spirit from the weight of the past.

This mudra stimulates a rejuvenating energy that helps clear your mind and direct it toward new, positive thoughts and possibilities.

Chakra: Solar plexus—3

Color: Yellow

Mantra: I AM THINE WAHE GURU
(I Am Thine, Divine Teacher Within)
Repeat mentally with each breath.

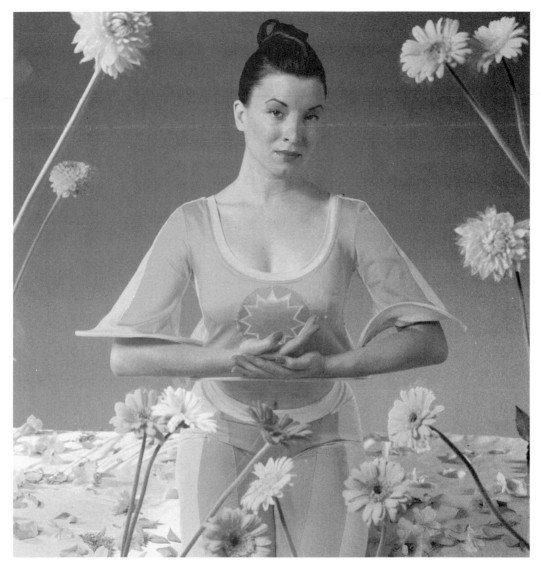

Sit or kneel with a straight back, elbows out to the sides, and bring your palms up to the level between your stomach and heart center. Palms are facing up, toward the sky, right hand resting in left. Upper arms are slightly away from the body. Breathe slowly and deeply. Think of the situation that burdens you and release that feeling with each exhalation. Now replace it with a positive affirmation—"I forgive myself"—and ask the Higher Power to erase any wrongs you may have done. BREATH: LONG, DEEP, AND SLOW. Practice for a few minutes and relax.

Mudra for Stronger Character

We all want to have strong, devoted, and loyal friends, life partners, and business associates. To attract people with these qualities into our lives, we must first develop these qualities within ourselves. Passing the moral tests of life—temptation, selfish motivation, and weak character—with which we are faced every day, makes us stronger in our character. Yet if we fail these tests, they will continue to present themselves. The practice of this pose will help you meet these challenges, build a strong character, and attract similar people into your life.

This mudra will change the metabolism of the mind and develop happiness of the spirit and personal power.

Chakra: Solar plexus—3
Third Eye—6

Color: Yellow, indigo

Mantra: HUMEE HUM BRAHAM
(Calling on the Infinite Self)
Repeat mentally with each breath.

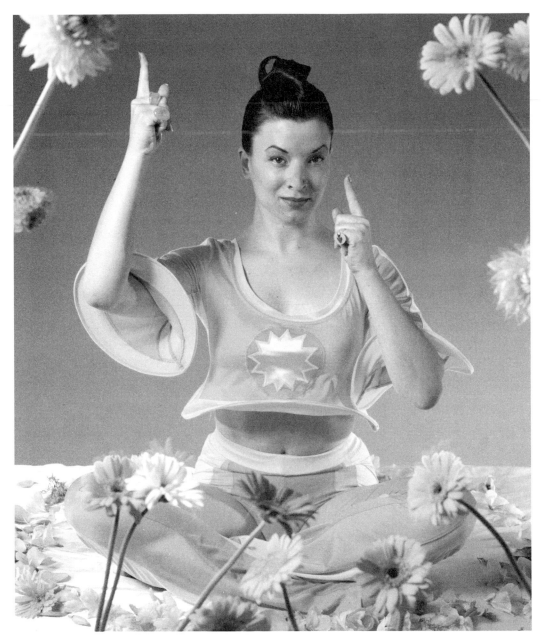

Sit with a straight back and hold your arms at your sides, your hands in re-laxed fists. Thumbs are outside, index fingers are straight. Lift your hands up, left hand at the level of your face and right fist slightly above your face. Hands are facing each other. Keep your eyes open and look forward. BREATH: LONG, DEEP, AND SLOW. Repeat for a few minutes and relax.

Mudra for Concentration

The power to concentrate magnifies your capacity to achieve your goals and attract positive experiences and people into your life. Mastering and directing your thoughts is the ultimate goal of concentration and is necessary for your spiritual evolution. You can learn to concentrate with practice.

This mudra helps you become calm while giving you the capacity to focus. It was used by saints and sages when they achieved samadhi, or the ultimate state of ecstatic meditation.

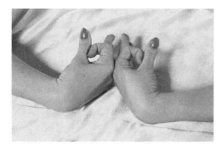

Chakra: Solar plexus—3
Heart—4
Third Eye—6

Color: Yellow, green, indigo

Mantra: AKAL AKAL AKAL HARI AKAAL
(Immortal Creator)
Repeat with each breath.

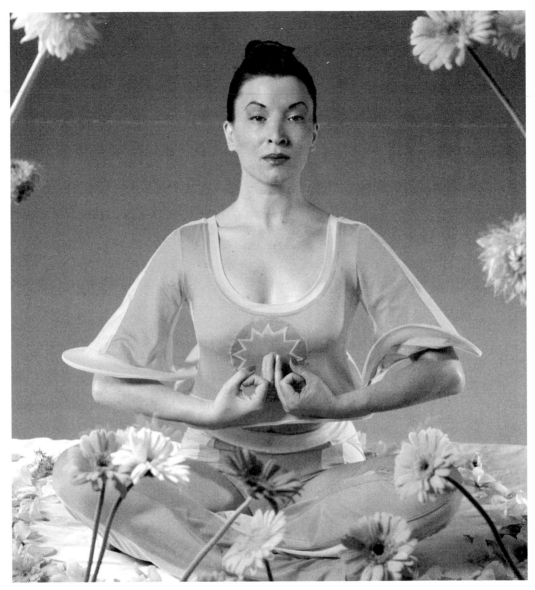

Sit in a comfortable position with a straight spine. Curl each thumb and index finger to create a circle, and keep the rest of the fingers straight, pointing up. Bring your hands in front of you just above your navel so that the up-stretched fingers are touching back to back, pointing toward the sky. Close your eyes and concentrate on your Third Eye area. BREATH: LONG, DEEP, AND SLOW. Still your mind and concentrate on a positive affirmation such as: "I AM the eternal light of the world. . . ."

Mudra for Overcoming Anxiety

Anxiety is a frequent reaction to the demands and stress of our lives. You can control your anxiety with regular daily practice of this mudra. You can also defuse a sudden anxiety attack by immediately practicing this mudra for a few minutes. You will instantly feel the difference and become more calm and centered.

This mudra creates its calming effect on your nerves by making a vortex of energy with each hand, which acts like a vent for your anxious energy.

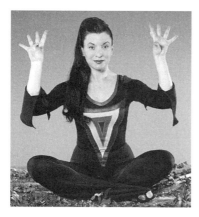 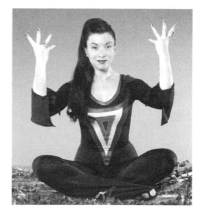

Chakra: Solar plexus—3
Heart—4

Color: Yellow, green

Mantra: HARKANAM SAT NAM
(God's Name Is Truth)
Repeat mentally with each breath.

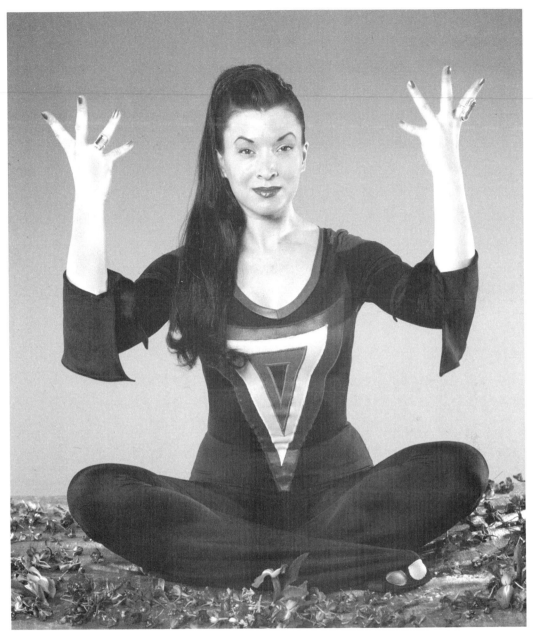

Sit with a straight spine. Bend your elbows and raise your arms so your upper arms are parallel to the ground and extended out to the sides. Your hands should be held at ear level, with fingers spread and pointing toward the sky. Rotate your hands back and forth, pivoting at the wrists. Continue for a few minutes and relax. BREATH: LONG, DEEP, AND SLOW.

Mudra for Transcending Anger and Preventing Headache

We all have the right to get upset at times, but harboring negative emotions is not productive or healthy. To help you transcend angry feelings and figure out how to express them appropriately, practice this mudra. Its immediate and powerful effect will help you channel your anger into a positive outcome or decision.

This mudra is also effective for preventing and curing headaches if you have a tendency to get them frequently.

This mudra works by creating an emotional equilibrium. The pressure points stimulated with your thumbs release anger and have an immediate calming effect.

Chakra: All Chakras

Color: All colors

Mantra: GOD AND I, I AND GOD ARE ONE
Repeat mentally with each breath.

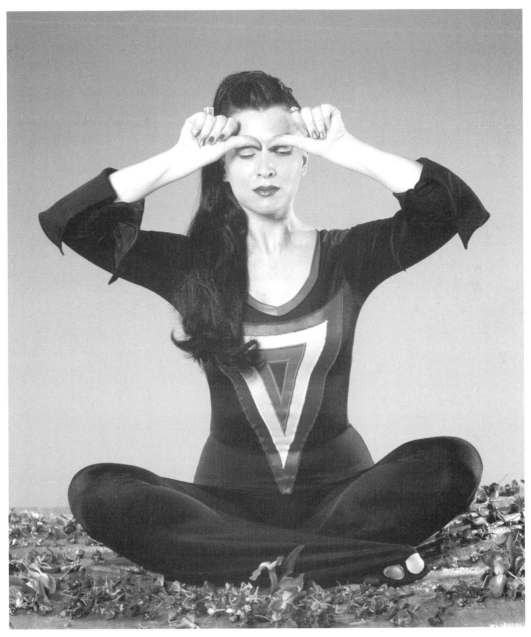

Sit in a comfortable position with a straight spine. Lift your hands to the level of your forehead. Make fists with the palms facing outward and keep the thumbs stretched pointing toward each other. Press the spot on your brow between your eyes and nose and focus your eyes at the tip of your nose. BREATH: LONG, DEEP, AND SLOW. Continue for three minutes and relax.

Mudra for a Sharp Mind

This mudra will help you make up your mind, particularly when you are faced with life-changing decisions. Regular practice of this mudra three times a day for three minutes will give you results in one week.

This mudra neutralizes the central part of the brain and gives you a sharp mind. The moving fingers are stimulating and massaging the meridian that affects your patience, emotional control, solar plexus, nerves, and vitality.

Chakra: Throat—5
Third Eye—6

Color: Blue, indigo

Mantra: HARA HARE HARI
(The Creator in Action)
Repeat mentally with each breath.

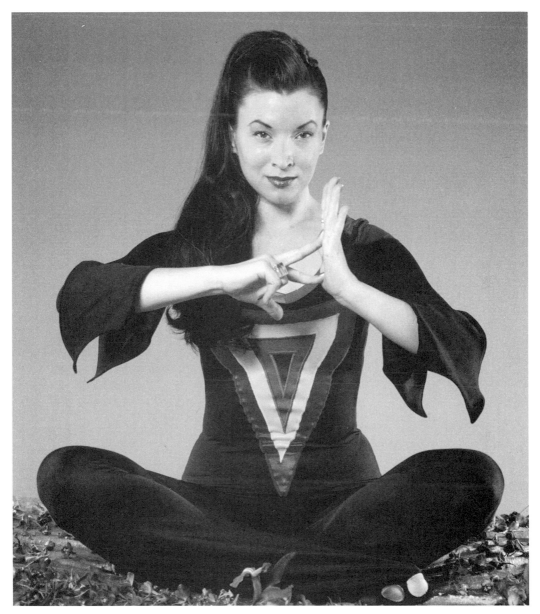

Sit with a straight back. Hold the left hand up as though to clap, then, with the index and middle fingers of the right hand, slowly and with strong pressure walk up the center of the left palm to the very tips of the middle and ring fingers. The left fingers should give in under pressure. Walk up and down a few times while concentrating on the movement of your fingers. BREATH: LONG, DEEP, AND SLOW.

Mudra for Patience

Patience is a virtue that everyone *can* develop. It is an important component of a happier, healthier life. Remember: In anything you do, after you have done your very best, relax and practice patience. Tell yourself that everything is happening at the right time, even when it seems to make no sense, and you will help make it so.

This mudra will help you transform your frustration and allow you to become more patient and tolerant. Your hands activate electric currents that channel healing energy to your nerves, thus calming you and helping you achieve patience.

Chakra: Third Eye—6
Crown—7

Color: Indigo, violet

Mantra: EK ONG KAR SAT GURU PRASAAD
(One Creator, Illuminated by God's Grace)
Repeat mentally with each breath.

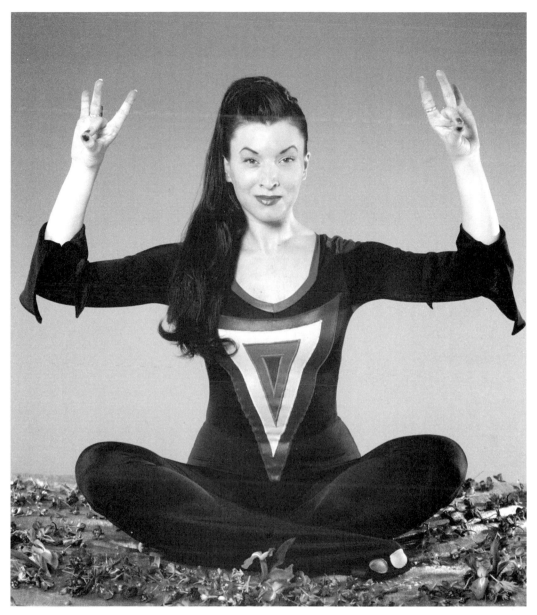

Sit with a straight back. Make circles with the tips of your thumbs and middle fingers, keeping the other fingers straight. Upper arms are parallel to the floor, elbows out to the sides. Your hands are at the level of your ears, fingers pointing toward the sky, palms facing front. BREATH: LONG, DEEP, AND SLOW. *Repeat for a few minutes and observe yourself becoming calmer and more patient with each breath.*

Mudra for Inner Security

Every day brings a new test of our self-confidence. Whenever you feel lost in this big world and overwhelmed by doubts, this mudra will restore your self-confidence and reinforce your sense of inner security. You must remember: You are never alone.

This mudra works in a positive and empowering way on the area of the brain that affects your sense of security.

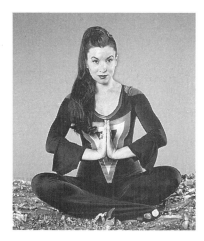 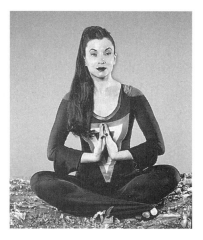

Chakra: Solar plexus—3
Heart—4

Color: Yellow, green

Mantra: AD SHAKTI AD SHAKTI
(I Bow to Creator's Power)
Repeat mentally with each breath.

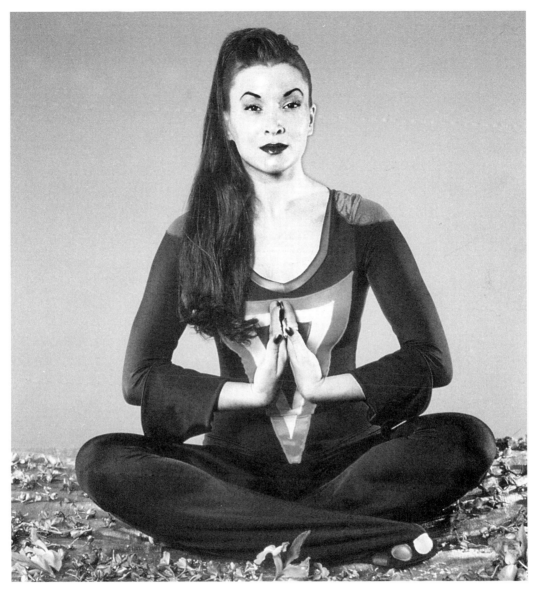

Sit with a straight spine and place your hands in a reversed prayer pose with hands touching back to back. Hold your hands in front of your heart. Imagine the energy moving from the bottom of your spine upward toward the top of your head. Hold this pose for one and a half minutes, then reverse the hands into a prayer pose with palms pressed together, thumbs against the chest. Hold for one and a half minutes. Repeat until you feel calm. BREATH: LONG, DEEP, AND SLOW.

Mudra for Calming Your Mind

A calm mind will give you the ability to center and focus your thoughts and so give you a tremendous capacity for success. The calmer your mind, the more you notice the unrest of others, and the faster you can achieve your goals.

This mudra stimulates your brain in a way that calms your mental activity and helps you control your focus.

Chakra: Solar plexus—3
Heart—4
Third Eye—6

Color: Yellow, green, indigo

Mantra: AKAL HARE HARI AKAL
(God Is Immortal in His Creation)
Repeat mentally with each breath.

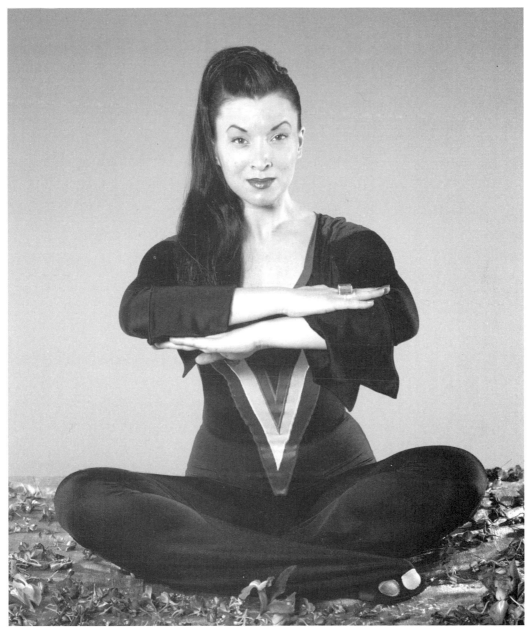

Sit with a straight back and cross your arms in front of your chest, elbows bent at a ninety-degree angle. Arms are parallel to the ground. Place the right palm on top of the left arm and the top of the left hand under the right arm. Fingers are together and straight. Hold this mudra and concentrate for a few minutes, then relax. BREATH: LONG, DEEP, AND SLOW.

Mudra for Keeping Up with Children

Children demand our constant attention, guidance, patience, and wisdom. It's not uncommon for parents to become overwhelmed by their sense of responsibility and to need some time to themselves. If you have only a few moments to get away from it all, it is most important to utilize that time efficiently to recharge yourself. This mudra can be practiced on the run, with just a few minutes to spare. It will do wonders for your ability to nurture your children.

This mudra will help you prepare to meet the needs of parenting on all levels.

Chakra: All chakras

Color: All colors

Mantra: AAD SUCH
JUGAAD SUCH
HAI BHEE SUCH
NANAK HOSEE
BHEE SUCH
(True in the Beginning, True in All Ages,
True at Present, True It Shall Ever Be)
Repeat mentally with each breath.

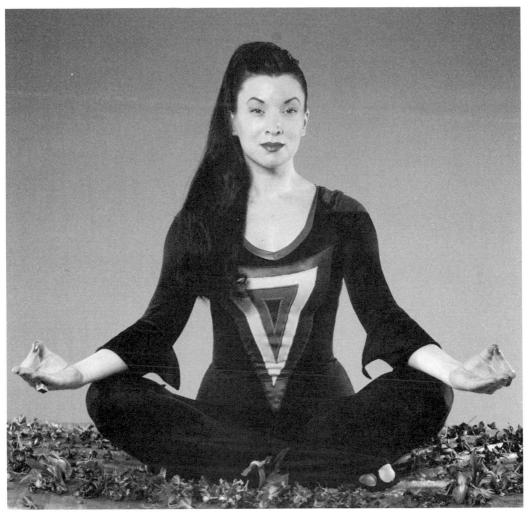

Sit with a straight spine. Make circles with the tips of the thumbs and index fingers. The other fingers are slightly relaxed but extended outward, while the hands rest on the knees. Concentrate on the Crown Chakra. BREATH: LONG, DEEP, AND SLOW. Continue for three minutes and relax.

Mudra for Taking Away Hardships

Challenges are an unavoidable part of life. Instead of seeing them negatively as struggles, ask yourself to form the intention to see them as perfectly planned opportunities for your spiritual growth. If you feel that you have had a few cases of "bad luck" and that you have become set in a pattern of pessimism and hardship, you may be creating the kind of energy that will attract such situations on an even greater scale. With this mudra, you can keep your mind and brain patterns on a positive frequency and attract positive energy and people into your life. Hardship and suffering can be replaced by power and strength, but it is your decision what your mindset is going to be. Regular practice will change your life.

This mudra works on the central channel of energy in your body and creates a vibration that takes away hardship and opens the way for positive energy.

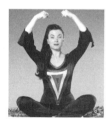 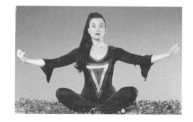

Chakra: Third Eye—6
Crown—7

Color: Indigo, violet

Mantra: HAR HARE GOBINDAY
HAR HARE MUKUNDAY
(He Is My Sustainer, He Is My Liberator)
Repeat mentally with each breath.

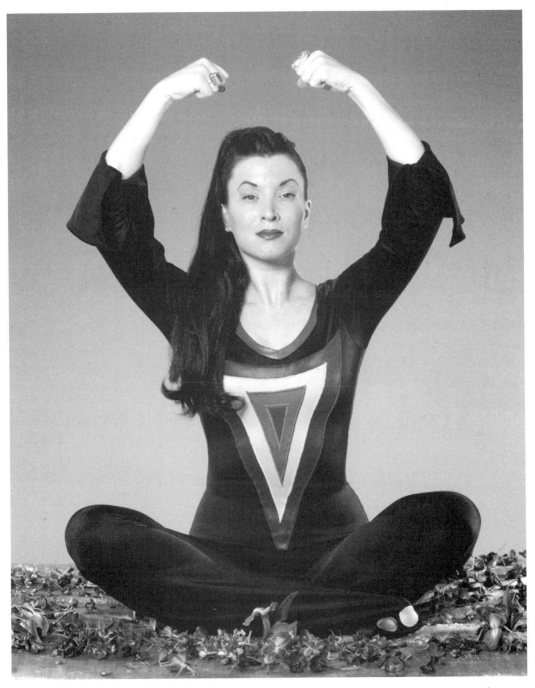

Sit with a straight back and make fists with both hands, thumbs outside. Begin swinging the arms backward in big circles, like a pendulum. First they go forward and up, and then they go back and down. BREATH: LONG, DEEP, AND SLOW. Continue for a few minutes. Relax and sit still.

Mudra for Efficiency

How many times have you been in a difficult situation and just did not feel sharp and focused enough to deal with it? Even a few minutes of doing this mudra before a meeting, exam, or confrontation will empower you to deal with the situation in the best possible way.

This mudra affects all the electric currents in your body, brings the entire nervous and glandular system into balance, and gives you razor-sharp efficiency.

Chakra: Heart—4
Third Eye—6

Color: Green, indigo

Mantra: ATMA PARMATMA GURU HARI
(Soul, Supreme Soul, the Teacher
in His Supreme Power and Wisdom)
Repeat mentally with each breath.

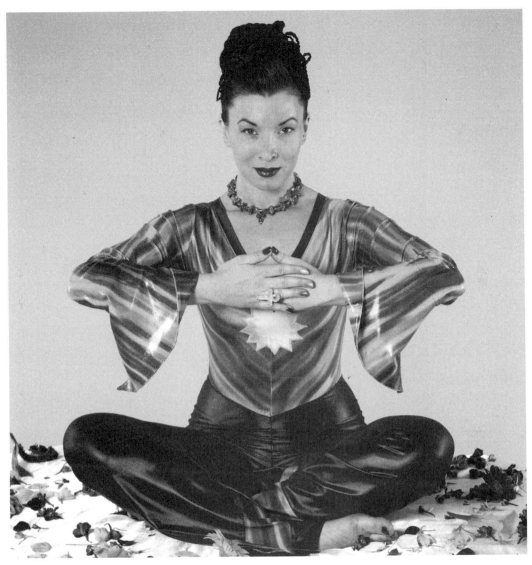

Sit with a straight spine. Bend your elbows, and raise your hands, palms facing your chest, so they overlap and touch at the level of your heart a few inches away from the body. The fingers of both hands are extended, palms facing the body. The palm of the right hand is placed over the back of the left. Press the thumb tips together and hold the hands and forearms parallel to the ground. BREATH: INHALE DEEPLY AND SLOWLY, HOLD THE BREATH FOR TEN SECONDS, AND EXHALE FOR TEN SECONDS. Wait ten seconds before inhaling again. Continue for a few minutes and relax.

Mudra for Tranquilizing the Mind

A calm ocean or sea . . . that's how our minds should be. It may take as long as a week of daily practice of this mudra to help you lead a calmer and more peaceful life, but it will work.

This ancient mudra was given by Buddha to his disciples to please and tranquilize their minds. It short-circuits worried, obsessive energy and replaces it with a calming, helpful vibration.

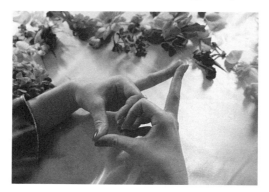

Chakra: Solar plexus—3
Heart—4
Throat—5
Third Eye—6

Color: Yellow, green, blue, indigo

Mantra: MAN HAR TAN HAR GURU HAR
(Mind with God, Soul with God,
the Divine Guide and His Supreme Wisdom)
Repeat mentally with each breath.

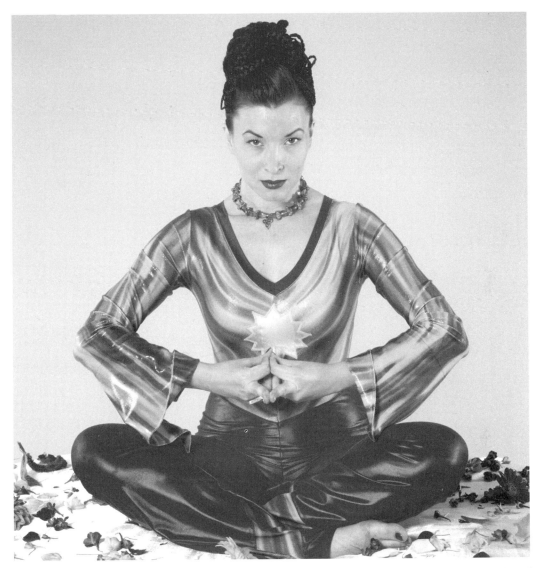

Sit with a straight spine and, with elbows bent, bring the hands up at the level of the navel. Bend the index fingers toward the palm and press them together along the second joint. Extend your middle fingers so that their finger pads are touching, pointing them away from your body. Curl the other fingers into your palm and touch the thumbs together at their tips, pointing toward you. Hold the mudra a few inches away from your body, elbows and hands held at the same level. BREATH: LONG, DEEP, AND SLOW. Continue for a few minutes and concentrate.

Mudra for Diminishing Worries

We all worry about something. Sometimes we worry out of habit, but there are times when we face truly difficult challenges. No matter what the magnitude of your problems, you can get a better perspective on them and take charge of your life with this mudra.

This mudra will reduce your worries.

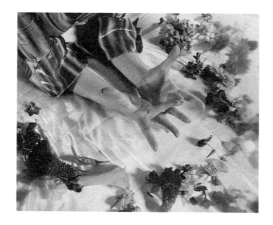

Chakra: Heart—4

Throat—5

Third Eye—6

Color: Green, blue, indigo

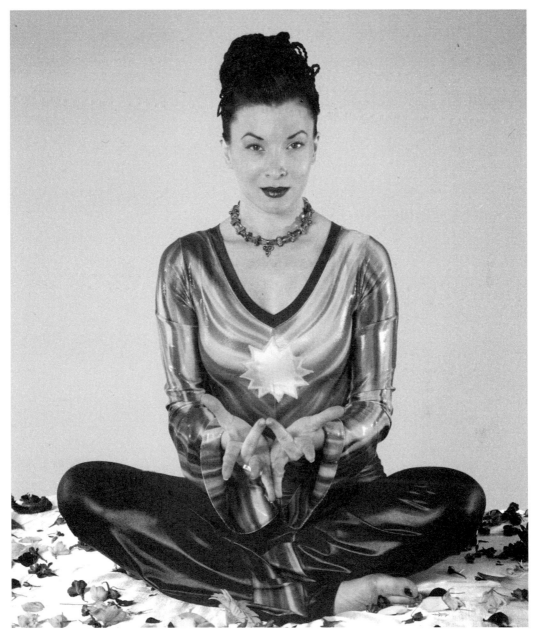

Sit with a straight back and bring your hands in front of your chest, palms facing up. The sides of the little fingers and inner sides of the palms are touching. Middle fingers are perpendicular to the palms, tips touching. Thumbs are extended away from the palms. Hold this mudra out of your chest. BREATH: IN-HALE LONG, DEEP, AND SLOW. *Continue for a few minutes and relax.*

Mudra for Removing Depression

For those times in life when everything seems bleak, if you can make an effort to do this mudra for only eleven minutes, your low feelings will diminish. Practice it once a day for a week and notice the difference. (If your depression has lasted for two weeks, see your doctor.)

The power of this mudra will help cure the worst depression. The position of your arms, hands, and fingers will send healing and positive vibrations to your brain centers, affecting your glands, which will help you remove this condition. You must practice for at least eleven minutes each time.

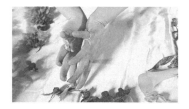

Chakra: Heart—4
Throat—5
Third Eye—6

Color: Green, blue, indigo

Mantra: HARI NAM SAT NAM
SAT NAM HARI NAM
(God Is Truth in Creation)
Repeat mentally with each breath.

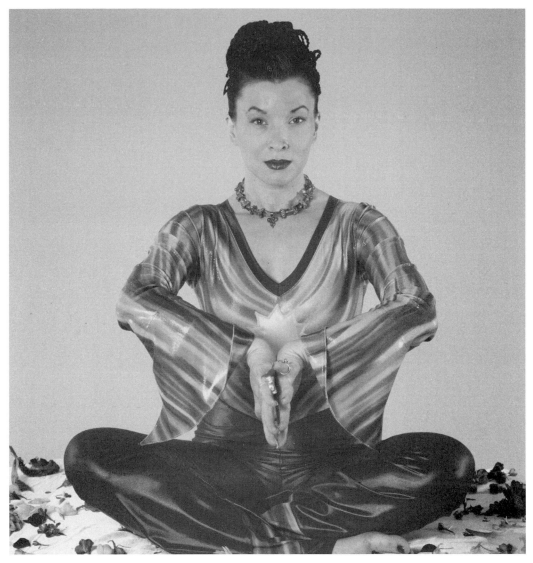

Sit with a straight spine. Stretch your arms in front of you, hands up at heart level. Put the backs of your hands together, with your fingers pointing away from your body, making sure that as many as possible of your knuckles touch. Your forearms are as parallel to the ground as possible, thumbs pointing down to the ground. This mudra creates a great deal of tension on the back part of your hands, but do not do this if you feel your muscles or tendons straining. BREATH: LONG, DEEP, AND SLOW. Continue for at least eleven minutes and feel the depression diminishing with each exhalation until it is gone.

Mudra for Self-confidence

A positive mind, body, and spirit are necessary for fulfilling your life's desires. Daily practice of this mudra will change your life and make you so self-confident that you will inspire others.

The power of this mudra adjusts the energy of the perception centers in your brain and improves your projection of positive energy. It also prevents self-defeating thoughts and actions.

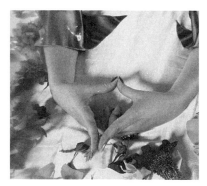

Chakra: Solar plexus—3
Third Eye—6

Color: Yellow, indigo

Mantra: EK ONG KAR SAT GURU PRASAD
SAT GURU PRASAD EK ONG KAR
(The Creator Is One That Dispels Darkness and
Illuminates Us by His Grace)
Repeat mentally with each breath.

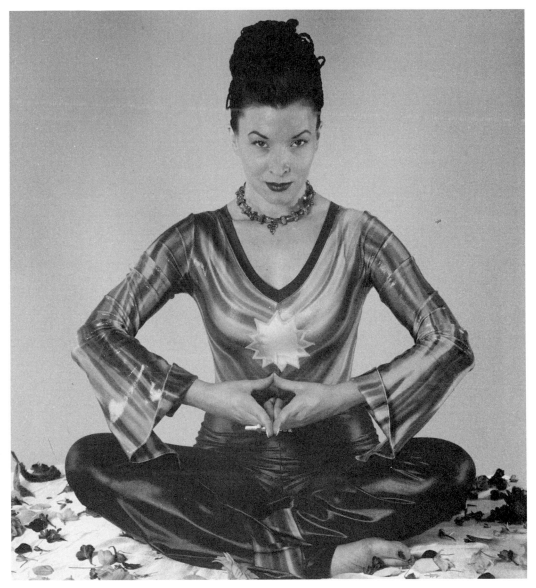

Sit comfortably with a straight spine. Lift your hands up to the level between your stomach and heart, elbows extended away from your body to the sides. Touch the middle knuckles of the last three fingers together. Point your index fingers out and away from your body, pads together. Point your thumbs back toward your chest as far as possible, touching each other from the last knuckle to the tip. Your thumbs are touching your body at the point of the solar plexus. BREATH: LONG, DEEP, AND SLOW. *Hold for a few minutes and relax.*

Mudra for Right Speech

Right speech is one of the five precepts, or virtues, that the Buddha taught as important for the spiritual path. Clear communication is essential for our survival. "Think before you speak" is good advice, but sometimes we are prompted to make impulsive responses and statements that harm ourselves and others. This mudra is your key for better speech and control of emotions. It will help you say what you wish so you can get what you want. You will gain friends and not enemies.

This mudra will make what you say consistent with your true intentions. It will also help you avoid saying things you don't mean.

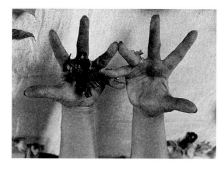

Chakra: Solar plexus—3
Throat—5

Color: Yellow, blue

Mantra: HAR DHAM HAR HAR
(God Is the Creator)
Repeat mentally with each breath.

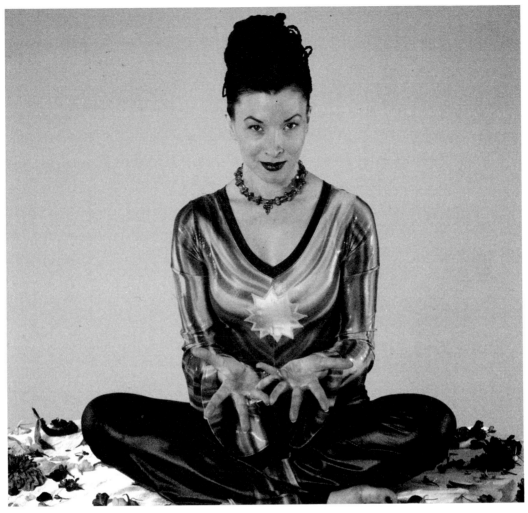

Sit with a straight spine. Relax your arms, keep your elbows at your sides, and bring your hands up in front of your stomach, palms open and flat, facing up. Spread your fingers gently and touch the tips of the ring fingers together. The right little finger is under the left little finger. Now concentrate and tense the thumb and the index fingers without moving the fingers. Hold for a few seconds and release. Now tense the thumb and the middle fingers, again without moving. Hold for a few seconds and release. Next, tense the thumb and the ring fingers. Hold and release. Lastly, tense the thumb and little fingers, hold for a few seconds, and relax. Repeat the cycle reversing the little fingers and relax. BREATH: LONG, DEEP, AND SLOW.

Mudra for Unblocking the Subconscious Mind

In our subconscious mind, we carry the memory and effects of positive and negative experiences. The energy of these negative memories—even if they are unconscious—can prevent us from reaching our true potential. You can tap into your subconscious memory, open it up, and clear it of these energy blockages with this mudra, which makes space for positive and powerful new energy to flow. Then you can refocus your thoughts and activities on fulfilling your life's mission.

This mudra will aid in the process of self-evaluation and transformation by stimulating the Third Eye points with the thumbs and fingers.

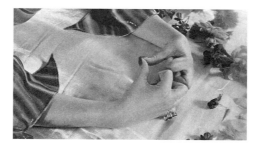

Chakra: Third Eye—6
Crown—7

Color: Indigo, violet

Mantra: ONG NAMO GURU DEV NAMO
(I Bow to the Infinity of the Creator, I Call on the
Infinite Creative Consciousness and Divine Wisdom)
Repeat mentally with each breath.

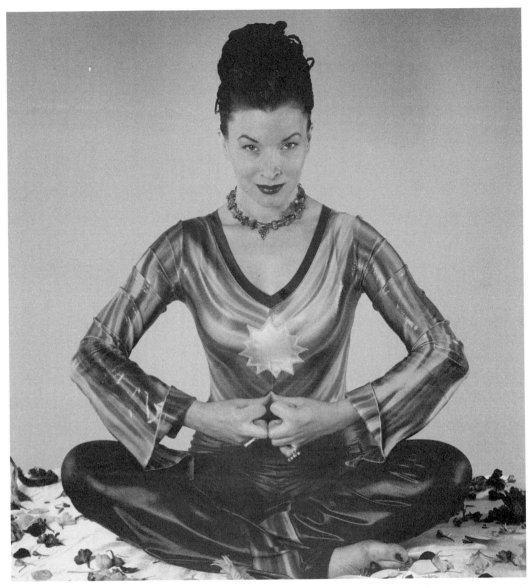

Sit with a straight spine. Relax and lift your arms up, out in front of you, elbows bent so your hands are in front of your stomach. Curl the fingers in so that the pads are touching the fleshy mounds at the base of the fingers. Thumb tips are together and the middle knuckles of the middle fingers are touching. No other fingers touch. Point your thumbs in a little toward the heart center. BREATH: LONG, DEEP, AND SLOW. Concentrate on the warmth between the thumbs. Continue for a few minutes and relax.

Mudra for Compassion

Each of us is born into a different set of circumstances and environment. Some people seem luckier than others, so we must always remember to count our blessings and feel compassion for others less fortunate. You can never truly imagine someone else's situation unless you have gone through a similar experience. The practice of being nonjudgmental and compassionate in our hearts is key to progress on our spiritual path and to sending good energy throughout the universe.

This mudra engages the heart center of compassion and the healing energy of the hands. It increases the circulation of blood to the brain, clears the mind, and improves concentration.

Chakra: Heart—4

Color: Green

Mantra: AKAL AKAL SIRI AKAL
(Timeless Is the One Who Achieves
Perfection of the Spirit)
Repeat mentally with each breath.

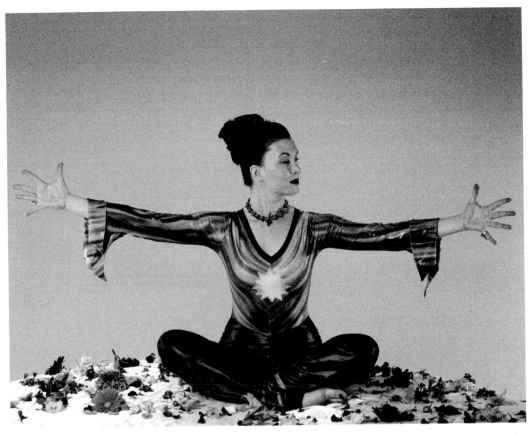

Sit with a straight spine. Extend your arms out to the sides parallel to the ground with the palms turned front. Stretch out the fingers and hold them still. Turn your head to the right side and back to the center four times, then to the left side and back to the center four times. Continue for a few minutes and concentrate on your heart center. Be aware of the energy in your hands. BREATH: INHALE LONG ONCE AS YOU MOVE YOUR HEAD TO THE RIGHT AND EXHALE LONG ONCE AS YOU MOVE YOUR HEAD BACK TO CENTER. REPEAT THE SAME FOR THE OTHER SIDE. Relax and sit still for a few minutes.

Sabrina Mesko started studying ballet at the age of three and was accepted into a professional company by the time she was a teenager. While recovering from a back injury, she discovered her passion for yoga. It became her daily routine, a discipline she would maintain throughout her career and continue for the rest of her life.

While touring the world as a Broadway dancer, Sabrina landed two starring roles on European TV and also began singing and composing music.

It was in New York that Sabrina had her first meeting with an Indian yoga master, Guru Maya. Her quest to combine spiritual enlightenment and expression through music soon took her to Los Angeles. While recording her own compositions, she began an intensive study of various spiritual teachings and meditation techniques of yoga, completed a four-year study of teachings with the world-renowned master Paramahansa Yogananda, and learned Kriya Yoga.

Sabrina also graduated with honors from the internationally known Yoga College of India and became a certified yoga therapist. She went on to study healing breath techniques with the master Sri Sri Ravi Shankar. She holds a bachelor's degree in Sensory Approaches to Healing, a master's in Holistic Science, and a doctorate in Ancient and Modern Approaches to Healing from the American Institute of Holistic Theology.

She felt compelled to develop her own unique yoga program, and while privately teaching, Sabrina saw the powerful transformation in her students' lives. The healing effects of her training would leave them in a state of calm, self-confidence, and joy.

Her fascination with the study of powerful hand gestures, mudras, led Sabrina to the world's only master of White Tantric Yoga, Yogi Bhajan. Recognizing her mission, Yogi Bhajan has entrusted Sabrina with the sacred mudra techniques and given her the responsibility to spread this ancient and powerful knowledge worldwide.

As a doctor of health theology, she is devoted to her work of healing through the power of music and dance. Sabrina combines all her experience and knowledge to create enlightening projects dedicated to bringing love, peace, and enlightenment to the planet.